Bill Young   5-2-46
Stanford Med School
Lincoln Hill

PRACTICAL
NEUROLOGICAL
DIAGNOSIS

Third Edition, Second Printing

PRACTICAL NEUROLOGICAL DIAGNOSIS

With Special Reference to the Problems of Neurosurgery

By

R. Glen Spurling, M. D.

Clinical Professor of Surgery (Neurosurgery)
University of Louisville School of Medicine
(On Leave of Absence)

CHARLES C THOMAS, PUBLISHER

301-327 East Lawrence Avenue
Springfield · *Illinois*

1 9 4 5

Published by CHARLES C THOMAS
301-327 EAST LAWRENCE AVENUE, SPRINGFIELD, ILLINOIS

Published simultaneously in Canada by
THE RYERSON PRESS, TORONTO

First Edition, February, 1935
Second Edition, October, 1940
Third Edition, September, 1944
Third Edition, Second Printing, August, 1945

Printed in the United States of America

PREFACE TO THE THIRD EDITION

RELATIVELY few changes have been made in the manuscript for the third edition; only the section on Myelography has been revised completely. This course was not occasioned by the exigencies of war or to limitations imposed upon me by the publisher, but rather to the belief that the book in its present form is as useful to students as anything I could write again.

R. GLEN SPURLING

Washington, D.C.
July 6, 1944

PREFACE TO THE SECOND EDITION

IN PREPARING the manuscript for the second edition my objectives have been threefold: *First,* to refrain from the temptation to enlarge the scope of the text and thus increase the size of the book. *Second,* to correct errors that crept into the first edition. *Third,* to include in the text as much new information as is consistent with my primary purpose of presenting to students and practitioners of medicine a *simple* account of the principles of neurological diagnosis.

My thanks are due primarily to reviewers of the first edition who kindly pointed out shortcomings. I have endeavored to profit by their criticism. I am deeply indebted to my former associate, Dr. F. Keith Bradford, for critically reviewing the manuscript and to Dr. Joseph C. Bell for many suggestions that led to a drastic revision of the section on Roentgen Diagnosis.

To Mr. Charles C Thomas, the publisher, I am always indebted for complete coöperation and helpful advice.

R. GLEN SPURLING

Louisville, Kentucky.
September, 1940

PREFACE TO THE FIRST EDITION

THIS VOLUME aims to present a simple account of the principles of neurological diagnosis. It is designed for students and practitioners who desire to become more proficient in the recognition of neurological disorders. It is not a glossary of symptoms and signs. Many duplicating diagnostic tests have been omitted. Only those which I have found, over a period of years, to be most useful are described. An attempt has been made to gather together from scattered sources data which explain the anatomical and physiological bases and the clinical interpretation of neurological symptoms and signs. In order to render the diagnostic study complete, chapters dealing with the cerebrospinal fluid and x-ray interpretation are included.

The outline for the neurological examination described is, with minor variations, used in many neurosurgical clinics. It is probably no better than many other synopses, unless, perhaps, it points more directly to a neurosurgical goal. It is, I believe, an entirely adequate guide in all organic disorders of the nervous system.

The field of organic neurology generally has not received the attention which it merits. Surgical lesions of the nervous system still too frequently come to the neurosurgeon in their final stages. If this condition is to be corrected, physicians and students generally must become more "neurologically minded." Toward this end I trust that this book may contribute a small part.

R. GLEN SPURLING

Louisville, Kentucky.
September 6, 1934

ACKNOWLEDGMENTS IN THE FIRST EDITION

THE INFORMATION contained in this book is the product of other minds—those of the past and present. My only claim to originality is in the arrangement and, in some instances, the interpretation of the material. The constant citation of authorities has been dispensed with because it encumbers a text primarily intended for students. A list of references has been appended at the end of Part I to indicate the authorities from whom much of the subject matter has been borrowed. To these authors I express my sincere thanks.

To the president of the University of Louisville, Dr. Raymond A. Kent, and to the dean of the Medical School, Dr. John W. Moore, I am thankful for placing at my disposal the facilities of that institution.

It would be impractical to mention the names of all my friends who have given encouragement and who have contributed valuable suggestions. In particular, I wish to express my debt to Dr. John F. Fulton and Dr. James B. Rogers, who critically reviewed the manuscript on the neurological examination. Drs. Franklin Jelsma, Malcom Thompson, George Wakerlin, and Clarence Bird kindly aided in many ways. Whatever merit of orthographic exactness this book possesses is due to the intelligent labor of my secretary, Miss Nellie Burdette.

The photographs were made by Dr. Clyde McNeill, a chore which he graciously undertook and for which I am appreciative. With few exceptions, the x-ray films were made by Dr. Joseph C. Bell from my own cases.

Miss Helen Woelfel made the drawings which speak for themselves. Some of the drawings were copied from textbooks and published articles and proper acknowledgment appears in the subtitles. To these authors and their publishers I am grateful for permission to reproduce their work.

The publisher, Mr. Charles C Thomas, has shown his devotion to the advancement of neurology by many publications. I am deeply appreciative of the advice and coöperation which he has generously extended during the preparation of the manuscript.

CONTENTS

PART I

THE NEUROLOGICAL EXAMINATION

OUTLINE OF
THE NEUROLOGICAL EXAMINATION*

Date.......................

I. GENERAL OBSERVATIONS:

Position of body, extremities and head.
State of consciousness, drowsiness, apathy, promptitude of responding.
General nutrition.
SKIN: Fine or coarse texture; pigmentation.
HAIR: Texture and distribution.
PERSPIRATION: General or localized, increased or decreased.
HEAD: Size, shape, dilated veins, exostoses, tenderness to percussion, cracked-pot resonance, auscultation.
NECK: Tenderness, rigidity.

II. CRANIAL NERVES:

1. OLFACTORY
   a. Subjective—Hallucinations of smell; loss or impairment of function.
   b. Objective—Response to test odors.

2. OPTIC
   a. Subjective—Failing vision; limitation of fields; hallucinations of light.
   b. Objective—Visual acuity; perimetry.
      Fundi: Shape, size, color of discs, lamina cribrosa, physiological cupping, engorged or tortuous veins, constriction or streaking of arteries, exudate, hemorrhage, choking.

3. OCULOMOTOR
4. TROCHLEAR
6. ABDUCENS
   a. Subjective—Diplopia.
   b. Objective—External ocular movements; nystagmus; ptosis; palpebral fissures.
      Pupils: Size, equality, regularity, reaction to light and accommodation.

5. TRIGEMINUS
   a. Subjective—Pain, paresthesias; numbness.

* Every neurological examination should be preceded by a carefully taken history. The story of the illness should be told as nearly as possible in the patient's own words, particular attention being paid to the chronological order of symptoms.

    b. Objective—*Sensory:* Anesthesia, hypesthesia, hyperesthesia; corneal reflex.
      Motor: Deviation of jaw; paralysis of temporal and masseter muscles.

7. FACIAL

    a. Subjective—Hyperacusis; taste disturbance; spasmodic contractions of facial muscles; disturbance of lacrimal and salivary secretions; asymmetry of face.

    b. Objective—*Motor:* Facial expression, nasolabial folds; inability to retract corner of mouth, close eye completely, or wrinkle forehead.
      Sensory: Taste on the anterior two-thirds of the tongue.
      Secretory: Lacrimal and salivary secretions.

8. ACOUSTIC

    A. *Cochlear:*

      a. Subjective—Impairment of auditory acuity; tinnitus.

      b. Objective—Tick of watch.
         Tuning-fork test:
           a. Rinne
           b. Weber
    Otoscopic examination.

    B. *Vestibular:*

      a. Subjective—Dizziness; unsteadiness of gait.

      b. Objective—1. Bárány test.
           2. See section on cerebellum.

9. GLOSSOPHARYNGEAL

    a. Subjective—Dysphagia.

    b. Objective—Taste on the posterior third of the tongue; pharyngeal reflex.

10. VAGUS

    a. Subjective—Regurgitation of fluids; difficulty of speech; projectile vomiting.

    b. Objective—Deviation of soft palate; pulse; laryngeal paralysis.

11. SPINAL ACCESSORY

    Paralysis of the sternocleidomastoid and trapezius muscles.

12. HYPOGLOSSAL

    Paralysis of the tongue.

III. CEREBRUM:

A. FRONTAL

a. Prefrontal Area:
   Cerebration; concentration; euphoria; change in habits, anosmia.

b. True Motor Area:
   Convulsions; paralysis.

c. Premotor Area:
   Clumsiness in skilled acts; forced grasping.

d. Motor Speech Area:
   Motor aphasia.

B. PARIETAL

Sensations of touch, pain, and temperature; astereognosis.

C. OCCIPITAL

Hallucinations of light; hemianopsia.

D. TEMPORAL

Acuity of hearing; hallucinations of smell; dreamy states; perimetric field defects; sensory aphasia.

E. CORPUS STRIATUM

Muscular rigidity; tremors; slowness of voluntary movements; change of emotional expression.

IV. CEREBELLUM:

Station; Romberg; gait; hypotonicity; nystagmus; dysarthria.

Finger-to-finger ⎫
Finger-to-thumb ⎪
Finger-to-nose   ⎬ Ataxia, asynergy
Heel-to-knee   ⎪
Past-pointing   ⎪
Adiadokokinesis ⎭

V. SPINAL CORD:

a. Subjective—Muscular weakness, local or general; difficulty in walking; dragging toe of shoe; stumbling or falling; sphincteric disturbances; changes in sensation, local or general; pain, fixed or radiating; abnormal sweating.

b. Objective—1. *Motor:* Range of muscular movement; contractures; atrophy; strength of muscles against resistance; tremors.

2. *Sensory:* Segmental sensory level: Pain, temperature, light touch, tactile discrimination; deep sensation (muscle, bone, joint, and vibratory sense).

VI. REFLEXES:

Superficial: Abdominal, cremasteric, Babinski, Chaddock, Oppenheim, and Gordon.

Deep: Biceps, triceps, knee- and ankle-jerks, radial periosteal, ankle-clonus.

VII. SUMMARY OF POSITIVE FINDINGS:

    a. Subjective—1.
                2.
                3. etc.
    b. Objective — 1.
                2.
                3. etc.

IMPRESSION:

CHAPTER I

HISTORY AND GENERAL OBSERVATIONS

In no other branch of medicine is it possible to build up a clinical picture so exact as to localization and pathological anatomy as in organic neurology. To do this, however, requires a certain diagnostic acumen usually not found in the student's armamentarium. In the first place, one must have a fairly exact general knowledge of neuro-anatomy and physiology. In the second place, the neurological examination must be made in an orderly manner if all the necessary details are to be elicited. In the third place, the novice must become familiar with a few special instruments and tests not ordinarily used in the general physical examination.

HISTORY

The neurological examination does not take the place of a general history and physical examination. It is merely a supplementary investigation. Symptoms referable to the nervous system are so frequently dependent upon general bodily disorders that it is essential for the examiner to have a clear understanding of the exact status of the patient's health.

The art of taking a neurological history is the same as elsewhere in medicine. The patient should be allowed to tell his story in his own words, in a logical sequence of details. It is important that each symptom be recorded in chronological order so that a clear conception of the progress of the disease may be had. Many patients will be incapable, for one reason or another, of giving a detailed history. In such circumstances, a relative or friend with whom he has been most closely associated offers the best solution. The examiner must understand clearly from the patient's story just what is meant by the term used in his symptomatology. For example, what may be a headache to one patient may be merely a fullness or neuralgia to another.

7

Almost invariably the patient will attribute the onset of symptoms to a "fall" or other trauma, even though the incident was of such minor importance as to have been forgotten until the onset of symptoms. Only occasionally is such a traumatic history significant.

After the patient has completed his own story, the examiner should elaborate by asking leading questions. The routine suggested is to follow the subjective part of the neurological outline step by step until every part of the nervous system has been covered. Negative as well as positive data should be recorded, for the negative data may be more important than the positive findings in arriving at a diagnosis. If the history is covered in this manner, the objective examination may be made without resorting to further questioning.

Certain symptoms deserve particular attention. *Headache* is by far the most common symptom of expanding lesions of the brain. Occasionally, the character and location of headache are of localizing value. Frontal tumors or abscesses, for example, usually cause bilateral frontal headache. Pituitary tumors produce characteristically bitemporal headache with pains radiating between the temples. The headache of cerebellar tumors may be limited to the suboccipital region, until hydrocephalus intervenes, when the pain becomes occipitofrontal or generalized.

Persistent recurring headaches should always be carefully investigated. Not infrequently they will be found to be due to increased intracranial pressure either from interference of cerebrospinal fluid circulation or from an increase in size of a space-occupying lesion. However, it must be remembered that brain tumors may attain tremendous size before increasing the intracranial pressure significantly; whereas, a small tumor blocking the cerebrospinal fluid pathways may produce fulminating pressure symptoms.

The headache of brain tumor is usually described as "deep," "expanding," "dull but unrelenting" and always "severe." Usually, there is no relief, night or day, without analgesic drugs. After such a bout of pain, which may have lasted for several days, the patient may suddenly become free of pain for a few hours or days, only to have it reappear with terrific intensity.

Severe headache occurs in many conditions other than brain tumors. The pain of migraine is perhaps as severe as any known variety of headache. It occurs characteristically in "attacks," and the pain is usually restricted to one-half of the head (hemicrania). Each attack lasts for hours or days, and when the pain is most severe, photophobia and other visual phenomena are prominent symptoms. Migraine usually appears early in life and has an hereditary background. Usually, the intensity of the attacks recedes after the fiftieth year.

Severe headaches are frequently associated with toxic and allergic disorders, hypertension, renal insufficiency and diseases of the accessory and nasal sinuses. Headaches due to histamine sensitization are a particularly prevalent and important group. The attacks of pain resemble in many respects those of migraine, being characteristically unilateral but not associated with visual disturbances.

Vomiting, especially when it occurs in conjunction with headache, is a most important neurological symptom. When a high degree of intracranial pressure exists, vomiting, not preceded by a sensation of nausea, may occur. There may be no relation to the eating of food. The vomitus may be expelled with explosive force (projectile vomiting).

Convulsions frequently occur in diseases of the brain whether the disease be inflammatory, toxic, degenerative or neoplastic in origin. It is important to distinguish clearly between convulsive seizures and syncope, vertigo, decerebrate rigidity, and the hysterical states. To do this careful history taking is invaluable. In analyzing a convulsion, it is most important to know whether the musculature was in tonic or clonic spasm; whether the attack was generalized or limited to one part of the body; whether it was preceded by an aura; whether the fit was followed by paralysis of some part of the body.

A generalized convulsion (grand mal) is preceded by an aura in about half the cases, starts with a cry and loss of consciousness, then a general tonic spasm which is soon replaced by a clonic spasm of all the voluntary musculature. There is usually cyanosis, biting of the tongue and incontinence of urine or feces. Headache often follows the attack and drowsiness for several hours is the rule.

Another frequent type of convulsion (psychomotor) not usually recognized as such, is characterized by periods of abnormal behavior with amnesia. As an example, the patient may, without explanation, leave a social gathering, wander aimlessly for an hour or more and awaken in his new surroundings without recollection of how he got there or what transpired in the meantime. These psychomotor attacks may follow patterns of great variety and are difficult to distinguish from the functional states on clinical findings alone.

A localized or focal convulsion (jacksonian) begins as a tonic spasm in the face, hand or foot and spreads upward or downward until one whole half of the body is involved. The tonic phase is usually followed by clonic movements in the same parts. This progressive motor discharge (jacksonian march) is not associated with loss of consciousness. For a few hours following the attack some degree of paralysis of the part first involved commonly occurs (Todd's paralysis). Such a convulsion indicates an irritative lesion of the contralateral motor cortex. Frequently, a sharply localized fit may progress to a generalized convulsion with loss of consciousness. Such focal attacks carry the same pathological implications as a true jacksonian convulsion. Sensory focal convulsions, following the exact pattern of the motor convulsions, are seen occasionally. They are due to an irritative lesion involving the contralateral sensory cortex.

General Observations

The student should train himself to observe every detail of a patient's appearance and demeanor from the moment of introduction. In neurological afflictions, this is particularly important, for it often happens that the most valuable information is obtained without realization on the patient's part that the examination has started. Does the patient stand erect without support? Does he assume a normal attitude in standing or walking? Is he alert and coöperative, drowsy or apathetic? Does he respond to questions promptly, or are his answers delayed and inaccurate? Is he oriented as to time and place? Does he show evidence of a recent loss or gain in weight?

Skin.—There is considerable variation in texture, pigmentation and dryness of normal skin. Only gross changes are significant. For instance, the skin in acromegaly is coarse and dry, while in pituitary insufficiency, it is fine and dry. Abnormal streaks of pigmentation (striae) on the lower abdomen and hips are common in pituitary disease associated with suprarenal dysfunction.

Overactivity of the sympathetic nerves to a part causes an excessively moist skin, while underactivity produces a dry skin. Often the level of a spinal cord lesion may be accurately determined by finding the line of demarcation between moist and dry skin. Below the level of the lesion the skin is dry, because the activity of the sympathetic fibers which supply the sweat glands is abolished. This test is readily made by gently stroking the skin with dry finger tips from below the suspected level upward. When the level of normal moisture is encountered, a distinct pull is felt on the finger tips.

Hair.—In pituitary disease, the texture and distribution of the hair over the entire body are altered frequently. Usually, the hair is coarse and dry. Axillary hair is scant or absent; pubic hair, if present, often takes on the distribution of the opposite sex. Since every expanding lesion of the brain may cause pituitary deficiency from increased intracranial pressure, such changes in the bodily hair are common occurrences.

Head.—A close scrutiny of the head is desirable in every case of suspected intracranial disease. In children, it is always important to determine the size and shape of the head, as interference with the circulation of cerebrospinal fluid may cause separation of the suture lines with progressive enlargement of the head. Normal circumferences of the head at various ages are shown in the following chart:

TABLE I*

AVERAGE CIRCUMFERENCE OF HEAD AND CHEST OF HEALTHY CHILDREN FROM BIRTH TO THREE YEARS

Age	Sex	Chest		Head	
		Inches	Cm.	Inches	Cm.
Birth	Boys	13.4	34.2	13.9	35.2
	Girls	13.0	33.0	13.5	34.3
6 months	Boys	16.5	41.9	17.0	43.2
	Girls	16.1	40.8	16.6	42.3
12 months	Boys	18.0	45.7	18.0	45.7
	Girls	17.5	44.5	17.5	44.5
18 months	Boys	18.7	47.8	18.6	47.5
	Girls	18.2	46.2	18.0	45.7
2 years	Boys	19.3	49.1	19.2	48.7
	Girls	18.8	48.0	18.6	47.5
2½ years	Boys	19.8	50.4	19.5	49.5
	Girls	19.3	49.1	19.0	48.2
3 years	Boys	20.3	51.5	19.8	50.4
	Girls	19.8	50.4	19.4	49.3

* After Holt and McIntosh, Diseases of Infancy and Childhood, Appleton, 1933.

The scalp should be examined closely for dilated veins. Asymmetrical dilated veins in the scalp may indicate the presence of an underlying meningioma or hemangioma. A nevus of the face or head may be accompanied by a vascular lesion of the brain.

Exostoses on the outer table of the skull may have no clinical significance. Yet an exostosis or what appears to be one may offer the only clue to the location of an underlying meningioma.

Tenderness to percussion or digital pressure is a common finding in brain tumors. This is particularly true of tumors involving the posterior fossa of the skull. In the acoustic neurinomas, suboccipital tenderness to pressure is almost always present.

"Cracked-pot" resonance (Macewen's sign) is common in children with cerebellar tumors or hydrocephalus from any cause. The sign is elicited by percussing the skull with the finger tips, thereby producing a note of "cracked-pot" quality.

When the hydrocephalus is acquired after the suture lines have thoroughly united, this sign is absent.

Auscultation of the head should be done in every case of suspected brain disease. A bell-type stethoscope is necessary. Intracranial aneurisms occur more frequently than is generally believed. Although patients usually complain of a noise in the head synchronous with the heart beat, auscultation may be the only means of verifying the diagnosis. Cortical hemangiomas and meningiomas may produce an audible bruit when the stethoscope is applied directly over the lesion.

Neck.—Tenderness and involuntary rigidity of the neck muscles are characteristic of inflammatory lesions of the meninges. These signs occur also in cervical cord tumors, cerebellar tumors, traumatic lesions of the brain and cervical spine, cervical arthritis and spondylitis. The test is made with the patient lying on the back in complete relaxation. The head is gently flexed on the chest until a definite involuntary resistance is felt in the neck muscles. Should flexion be continued beyond this point, pain of varying intensity occurs.

At this point, it may be stated that the neurological examination of infants and young children offers an especially difficult problem. These little patients have no way of registering their complaints other than by crying, fretting, refusal of food, drowsiness and similarly indefinite signs. Nor is the mother's account of the illness likely to be more helpful. In approaching the diagnostic problem in these patients, one must take a purely objective view, much the same as an analysis of an experimental animal.

All too frequently an infant or child will be treated week after week for a supposed gastro-intestinal disorder, and finally when blindness supervenes, the first suspicion of a primary neurological disorder will be aroused. Also, it is an established observation in pediatrics, that the average case of meningococcus meningitis in infancy is first recognized in the second week of the illness!

If the profession would but recognize that much the same types of neurological disorders occur in the infant and child as in the adult, the incidence of correct diagnoses would be tremendously improved. The prevalent conception that tumors of the brain are of rare occurrence in the young is gradually being dissipated. As a matter of record, the incidence of brain tumor in the second decade of life is almost as high as in any decade in the natural life span.

CHAPTER II

THE CRANIAL NERVES

Many of the steps in the examination are divided into two parts: *Subjective,* what the patient tells the examiner, and *objective,* what the examiner finds out from his own observations. This method is useful for the trained neurologist as well as the novice, for it keeps the important complaints before the recorder in an orderly fashion.

1. THE OLFACTORY (*sensory*)

ANATOMY.—The end-organs of smell are located in the superior part of the nasal mucous membrane. They are composed of bipolar sensory cells, the ciliated distal portions of which reach the surface of the epithelium. The central processes are unmyelinated fibers which are grouped together in small bundles and constitute the olfactory nerve. These bundles pass through the cribriform plate of the ethmoid bone and enter the olfactory bulb. The bulbs lie in contact with the cribriform plate. From the olfactory bulbs, the neurons of the second order form the olfactory tracts which have their cortical center in the uncinate and hippocampal gyri of the temporal lobes. Each bulb receives fibers from the other by way of the anterior commissure.

CLINICAL.—Hallucinations of smell are often present in tumors or abscesses involving the deeper or inferior portions of the temporal lobe. Unpleasant odors like those of burning rubber, kerosene, or rotting flesh are the rule, but pleasant odors may occur. These hallucinations come in attacks during which the patient is often out of contact with his environment. Such an attack (uncinate fit) may constitute the aura of a major convulsion or may constitute the entire episode (convulsive equivalent).

Partial or even complete loss of the sense of smell (anosmia) is most often due to inflammatory diseases of the nasal mucosa and accessory air sinuses or to atrophic rhinitis. Complete

15

anosmia is very frequently a permanent sequela to skull fracture involving the cribriform plate of the ethmoids. Meningiomas of the olfactory groove and other tumors or abscesses
involving the frontal lobe produce bilateral or unilateral
anosmia. It must be remembered that a patient with anosmia
will often complain that he does not taste since the flavors of
foods other than salt, bitter, sweet and sour depend not upon
taste, but upon olfactory sense. In a suspected frontal lobe
lesion the presence of bilateral or unilateral anosmia may be a
very helpful sign in arriving at a diagnosis.

Each nostril is tested separately, the other being closed by
digital pressure. Highly volatile test substances are to be avoided as they irritate other sensory nerve endings, particularly
those of taste. Finely ground coffee gives a most satisfactory
test odor. The patient sniffs the test substance and reports any
perception of smell. If the odor is perceptible, then he is asked

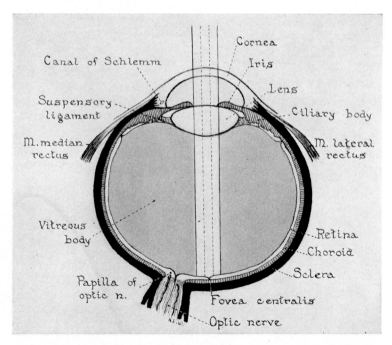

FIG. 1. Cross section diagram showing the principal structures of the eye.
(After Homans)

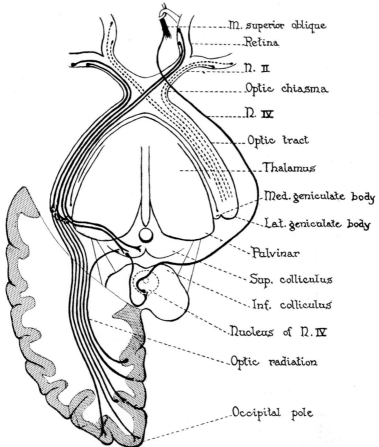

M. superior oblique

Retina

n. II

Optic chiasma

n. IV

Optic tract

Thalamus

Med. geniculate body

Lat. geniculate body

Pulvinar

Sup. colliculus

Inf. colliculus

Nucleus of n. IV

Optic radiation

Occipital pole

FIG. 2. Diagram of the optic pathways. (Modified from Ranson.)

to identify it. The appreciation of an odor, even without identification, is sufficient to exclude anosmia.

2. THE OPTIC (*sensory*)

ANATOMY.—The visual pathways are composed of the retinae, optic nerves, primary visual centers, optic radiations, and secondary or cortical visual centers.

Retina.—In embryonic life, the retina develops from the neural tube which forms the brain. It is composed of visual cells, neuroglia, and ganglion cells. The visual cells are bipolar, and their external process forms the rods and cones which act as visual receptors. The other process connects through an intermediate neuron with the ganglion cells, whose fibers in turn form the optic nerves. The ganglion cell fibers all converge at the posterior pole of the retina and form the optic disc (nerve head). At a point about 3 mm. to the temporal side of the optic disc is the macula (fovea centralis) where the most highly developed end-organs of sight are found, and likewise the most acute vision (Fig. 1).

The inner layers of the retina are supplied with blood from the central retinal artery which enters the eyeball through the optic nerve. The outer layers of the retina receive their blood supply from the choroidal circulation.

Optic Nerve.—The point of exit from the eyeball of the collected nerve fibers is at the optic disc. As the individual fibers pass through the meshes of the sclera, a sieve-like structure is formed called the lamina cribrosa. Since there are no end-organs of sight in this area, light rays striking directly upon the nerve head go unrecognized, thereby producing the blind spot.

The optic nerve enters the cranium through the optic foramen and unites with its fellow of the opposite side to form the optic chiasm. In the chiasm, a partial decussation of fibers from the two sides takes place (Fig. 2). Behind the decussation, fibers from both retinae are contained in each optic tract; each tract receives the fibers from the lateral half of the retina of its own side and those from the mesial half of the opposite side. From the chiasm, the tract passes around the thalamus and ends in the lateral geniculate body and the superior colliculus of the corpora quadrigemina. The superior colliculus is a reflex center, and the fibers of the optic nerve which terminate in it provide a mechanism for optic reflexes.

Optic Radiations.—The visual impulses brought to the lateral geniculate body are relayed to the cerebral cortex and give rise to visual perceptions. These fibers, called the optic radiations, pass backward through the posterior portion of the internal capsule to the visual cortex in the occipital lobes of the brain (Fig. 2). The fibers of the optic radiation which leave the lateral geniculate body bend sharply upon themselves to pass below the temporal horn of the lateral ventricle. Thence, they are directed backward through the white matter of the temporal lobe into the occipital lobe. Lesions of the temporal lobe often involve this part of the optic radiation and cause blindness in the opposite field of vision.

CLINICAL.—Symptoms referable to the optic nerve are among the most common for which the patient with an expanding lesion of the brain consults a physician.

Irritative lesions of the visual cortex may cause hallucinations of light. The patient will complain that with his eyes closed or open, a ball of fire floats into his field of vision and bursts, sending out millions of sparks. Flashes of light (like sheet lightning) are another fairly common form of visual hallucinations.

Destructive lesions in any part of the visual pathway or cortex cause defects in the field of vision. Such defects are often noticed by the patient. It is not uncommon for him to complain of bumping into people on his right side, because he does not see them (right homonymous hemianopsia), or that he cannot see well to either side without turning his head (bitemporal hemianopsia).

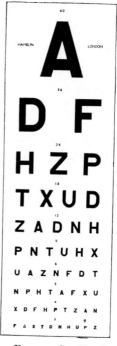

FIG. 3. Snellen's Test Types. The usual style of chart for testing visual acuity.

Acuity of Vision.—As indicated above, the most sensitive portion of the retina is in the region of the macula. When a distant image is desired, the eyes are so fixed that the light rays fall directly upon this region. This is called direct vision. In testing for direct vision, a range of 20 feet is selected, since rays of light from this distance are nearly parallel. A Snellen's test chart is used (Fig. 3). Each eye is tested separately. The patient should read the top line at

200 feet, the second line at 100 feet, the third line at 70 feet, the fourth line at 50 feet, the fifth line at 40 feet, the sixth line at 30 feet and the seventh line at 20 feet. At 20 feet, a person with normal direct vision should read the seventh line without difficulty. Therefore, the minimal normal vision is expressed as 20/20. Should he be unable to read any line below the third, his vision would be 20/70. Errors of refraction should have been corrected before the acuity tests have neurological significance. A patient losing his vision from intracranial disease will usually not be improved with glasses.

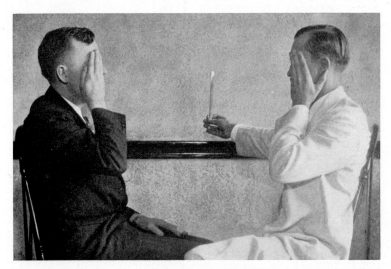

Fig. 4. Showing the position of the examiner and patient during a rough examination of the visual fields.

Field of Vision.—Gross defects in the visual fields can readily be detected by a very simple examination (Fig. 4). The examiner and patient are seated facing each other, the chairs being about 2 feet apart. When testing the left eye, the right eye is covered by the patient's right hand, while the examiner covers his left eye. The patient fixes his left eye on the pupil of the examiner's right eye, care being taken that the two heads are on the same level and in the same position. The test object consists of a ball of white absorbent cotton about 3 mm. in diameter at-

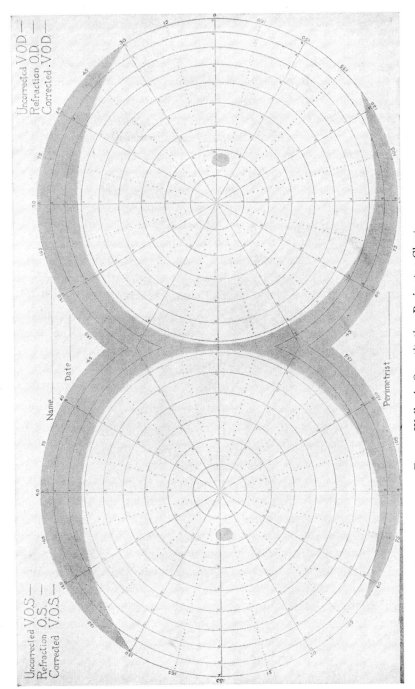

Uncorrected V.O.D —
Refraction O.D. —
Corrected V.O.D —

Name —— Date ——

Perimetrist ——

Uncorrected V.O.S —
Refraction O.S. —
Corrected V.O.S —

Fig. 5. Walker's Quantitative Perimeter Chart.

tached to an ordinary metal probe or to a wooden applicator. The test object is moved on a straight line midway between the patient and the examiner. The field of vision is outlined by moving the test object from the periphery on a vertical and horizontal plane, i.e., laterally, mesially, upward and downward. Assuming that the examiner knows his own field of vision, any abnormalities from his own may be readily found. The degree of limitation is calculated, using the examiner's field as the normal. The blind spot can be identified easily in this manner. Also, any abnormal blind spots (scotomata) may be mapped out.

For an accurate form, or color field of vision, the arc or screen perimeter is indispensable. If the reader has access to one of these instruments, he is advised to perfect himself in the technique of its use, as there are few instruments of precision more valuable in neurological diagnosis. The extent of the normal field on the arc perimeter at the usual perimetric distance is shown in Fig. 5. A discussion of color fields is not included here, since they have a relatively limited use in neurological diagnosis. Quantitative perimetry (i.e., the use of three white test objects, 1 mm., 5 mm., and 10 mm.) answers most needs.

Pathological Changes in the Visual Fields.—Pressure upon the visual pathways at any point from the visual centers in the occipital lobe to the retina, produces certain changes of function in the involved fibers which are reflected in and may be recognized by examining the fields of vision (Fig. 6).

A lesion pressing upon the left optic nerve may destroy all the fibers to both halves of the retina, and the resulting visual defect would be complete blindness in the left eye (Fig. 6A).

If a lesion presses upon the middle portion of the optic chiasm (pituitary tumor) it may destroy all the decussating fibers which supply the inner or nasal halves of the retinae, and thereby produce loss of vision in the outer or temporal halves of the field of both eyes, a condition called *bitemporal hemianopsia*

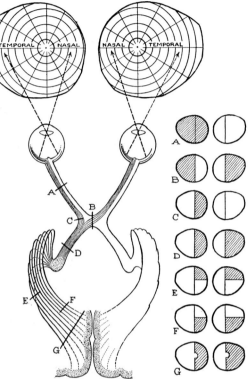

FIG. 6. The Optic Pathway, showing how lesions at various points will be exhibited in the Fields of Vision upon perimetric examination. The shaded areas, in the small perimetric fields on the right, correspond to the lesions marked on the left-hand figure as follows: A.—Total blindness in the left eye. B.—Bitemporal hemianopsia. C.—Nasal hemianopsia in the left eye. D.—Right homonymous hemianopsia. E. and F.—Right upper and lower quadrantal homonymous hemianopsias respectively. G.—Right homonymous hemianopsia with preservation of central vision. (Homans)

(Fig. 6B). Here, too, the field defect may be complete or incomplete.

A lesion at the level of the optic chiasm, which destroys only the outer (non-decussating) fibers of the left optic tract, leaving intact the inner (decussating) fibers, will produce loss of function in the temporal half of the retina of the left eye, thereby producing blindness in the nasal field, i.e., nasal hemianopsia in the left eye (Fig. 6C).

When one-half of a visual field is absent, the defect is called hemianopsia. If a lesion destroys the left optic radiation or the left visual cortex, loss of function in the left halves of both retinae and, consequently, blindness in the right field of vision of both eyes results. This condition is known as right *homonymous* hemianopsia (Fig. 6D). Obviously, if only a part of the fibers of this tract were involved, the loss of vision in the right homonymous fields would be incomplete. Such conditions are usually spoken of clinically as right homonymous visual field defects.

If a lesion involves only a portion of the optic radiations in their course through the temporal lobe to the occipital lobe, the defect produced in the visual fields takes the form of quadrant homonymous hemianopsia. If the lesion involves the outer fibers of the left radiations, the defect produced will be right upper quadrant homonymous hemianopsia (Fig. 6E).

If the lesion involves the inner fibers of the radiations, the field defect is called right lower quadrant homonymous hemianopsia (Fig. 6F).

If the lesion destroys the visual cortex of the pole of the left occipital lobe, the resultant field defect is right homonymous hemianopsia with preservation of central vision. The explanation for the preservation of central vision is that the fibers of the macula are not destroyed, since the macula has a wide cortical representation extending on the mesial surface of the hemisphere down to the corpus callosum (Fig. 6G).

The reader will find it profitable to study carefully Fig. 6. If he wishes to indulge in some mental gymnastics, cover the visual charts on the right side of the drawing and figure what field defects would result from the lesions as indicated in the visual pathways.

Examination of the Fundus.—When Helmholtz in 1851 invented the ophthalmoscope, he gave to medicine one of its most useful instruments of precision. This instrument has been epoch making in ophthalmology. In general medicine and neurology, its value is incalculable. The modern indirectly lighted electric ophthalmoscope is an instrument which the novice can learn to operate in a proficient manner with a few hours of practice, and its cost is reasonable. One of these instruments should be a part of every student's and practitioner's equipment.

How does one justify this statement? Because by study of the fundus of the eye, certain information can be obtained during life relative to the eye itself, the brain, the blood vessels, the kidneys, and certain systemic infections which would remain a matter of conjecture were it not for this instrument.

Technique of Ophthalmoscopy.—The use of mydriatics to dilate the pupil for examination of the fundus is a time-

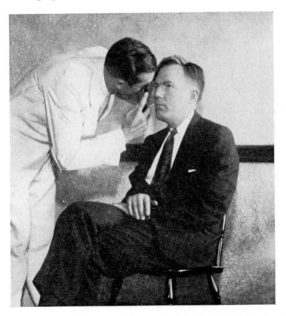

FIG. 7. Correct position of the examiner and patient during the ophthalmoscopic examination of the right eye.

honored custom. For the neurologist, this custom is the source of great annoyance, because it deprives him of information relative to the pupil which may be of great diagnostic importance. Except in rare instances, the use of mydriatics is not only unnecessary but undesirable. If the patient is placed in a darkened room for a few minutes before starting the examination, a very satisfactory view of the fundus can be obtained. The ciliospinal reflex (page 38) may be utilized to dilate the pupil for ophthalmoscopic examination when a darkened room is not available. The examiner or an assistant pinches gently the skin of the patient's neck and a prompt temporary homolateral dilatation of the pupil will follow. This period of dilatation is usually sufficiently long to permit a satisfactory cursory examination of the fundus. Opacities in the cornea, aqueous humor, lens, or vitreous humor may hinder or even preclude a satisfactory examination of the fundus. Fortunately, such abnormalities are but rarely met with in neurological cases.

The examination may be made with the patient standing, sitting or recumbent. The patient is told to look directly forward and not to move the eyes. It is often useful to flash the light of the ophthalmoscope in the direction he is asked to fix his gaze (Fig. 7). When examining the patient's right eye, the observer holds the ophthalmoscope in his right hand and uses his right eye; the left eye is examined with the observer holding the instrument in his left hand and using his left eye. The ophthalmoscope is brought directly in front of the patient's eye as closely as possible; not more than one inch should separate the eyes of the patient and observer.

The lens dial is set at zero. If there are no refractive errors in the eyes of the patient or examiner, the fundus will be in clear view at this lens setting. The novice often finds it difficult to relax his accommodation and it may be necessary in the beginning to correct for it by rotating a concave (minus) lens into place. Errors of refraction in either the patient's or observer's eyes may be corrected for by the use of the lenses in the ophthalmoscope. When the instrument is held properly, rotation of the lenses is a simple matter and disturbs neither the observer nor the patient.

Always begin the examination by looking for the optic disc, this being the most prominent landmark. If the disc is not found promptly, follow the vessels as they converge to the central artery and vein.

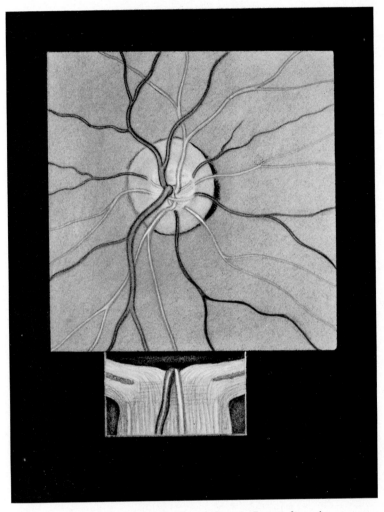

Fɪɢ. 8. Drawing of the normal fundus of the eye. Insert shows in cross section the optic disc, central artery and vein, and the physiological cup.

The Normal Fundus.—There are a great many variations of detail in the normal fundus. The disc is usually circular but may be oval in form. It is light pink in color, the temporal margin being paler than the nasal. The margin on the temporal side is usually sharply defined, while the nasal margin is more obscure in definition. Pigmentation around the temporal border or even around the entire disc is usually seen; this is the pigmented choroidal layer around the aperture through which the optic nerve passes. In the center of the disc is seen a depression caused by separation of the nerve fibers as they spread over the retina. This depression is called the physiological cup (Fig. 8). The cup varies greatly in size, rarely under normal conditions occupying more than one-half of the disc. At the bottom of this physiological excavation, one frequently sees a "sieve-like" arrangement of gray spots called the lamina cribrosa, produced by the optic nerve fibers passing through the sclera.

The central artery and vein of the optic nerve emerge from the disc at the physiological cup, and immediately divide into the superior and inferior divisions. Each of these vessels soon divides and subdivides. The appearance of the arteries and veins is quite dissimilar, the arteries being smaller in caliber and their course much straighter than the corresponding vein. Normally, the arteries appear to be hollow, because of a light streak running along the center. This is produced by the illumination from the ophthalmoscope striking the rounded surface of the vessel, thereby causing reflection of light. The same light reflex, but much less marked, is observed on the veins.

The retina is transparent. The color of the background comes from the choroidal vessels and the pigment of the choroid. The region of the macula lutea is often indistinguishable in the normal fundus. It is located about 2 disc diameters to the temporal side of the entrance of the optic nerve. It is devoid of visible vessels and usually somewhat darker than the rest of the fundus.

Because of the many minor variations in the normal fundus, considerable experience is necessary to distinguish between the normal and abnormal.

Papilloedema (choked disc, optic neuritis).—The optic nerve has as its covering a prolongation of the membranes of the brain. The dura, when it reaches the optic foramen, splits, and the outer layer forms the periosteal lining of the orbit, and the inner layer forms the external sheath of the optic nerve. Beneath this sheath and immediately surrounding the nerve,

lies the pia-arachnoid. The subarachnoid space of the brain
with its cerebrospinal fluid is thus continuous around the optic
nerve. The central vein of the retina, in its course to empty into
the superior ophthalmic vein, traverses the subarachnoid space
of the optic sheath.

Papilloedema is believed to be produced by venous congestion of the optic disc and retina, from compression of the
central vein of the retina by a distended subarachnoid space
of the optic sheath. The distention of the sheath is almost
always secondary to increased intracranial pressure.

The ophthalmoscopic picture is as follows: At first, the disc
is redder and the veins fuller than normal; the nasal, upper
and lower margins of the disc are blurred; the lamina cribrosa
is no longer distinguishable. As the edema increases, the physiological cup becomes obliterated, and the nerve head is elevated
above the level of the adjacent retina; the vessels become more
engorged and tortuous. As the congestion becomes greater,
elevation of the disc becomes more pronounced, and the margins cannot be identified; the vessels over the disc may be
embedded in exudate; fan-shaped hemorrhages may appear
over the retina or disc, and the surrounding retina becomes
edematous (Fig. 9). Unless the cause is relieved, the condition
progresses to secondary optic atrophy. As atrophy ensues, the
swelling becomes less; the disc grows paler and less vascular,
the arteries thickened and constricted, and the veins tortuous
but no longer engorged. Finally, the disc is snow white with
blurred edges.

During the early stages of papilloedema, vision may not be
impaired, but sooner or later, if the process remains unabated,
visual failure sets in and blindness results. During the first
phase of visual loss, the fields become concentrically constricted, and the blind spot is enlarged. In later stages, scotomata appear, and constriction of the field continues. Usually,
peripheral vision is lost first and central vision last.

The recognition of early stages of papilloedema would save
many patients from a life of blindness. All too frequently, patients, already blind as a result of an operable tumor or abscess

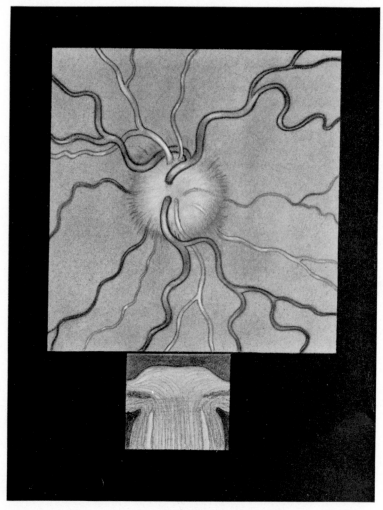

FIG. 9. Drawing of a moderately advanced "choked disc." Insert shows a
cross section of the swollen optic disc.

of the brain, seek surgical relief. It is only through the widespread intelligent use of the ophthalmoscope by the profession
that these catastrophies can be prevented.

The degree of papilloedema may be measured by means of
the series of lenses in the ophthalmoscope. The structures on

the surface of the disc are first brought into focus. To obtain a clear view of the elevated surface of the disc, a plus (convex) lens is usually required. When a sharp focus is obtained, the number of the lens used is noted. (As an example, let us say a +2 lens is required.) The next step is to obtain a sharp focus on the vessels of the retina well away from and to the outside of the disc, and the lens used in this step is noted. (Suppose a —2 lens is required.) The difference in the lens used in the first and second steps represents the amount of swelling at the nerve head expressed in diopters. (A +2 lens for the disc and a —2 lens for the retina equal 4 diopters elevation of the nerve head itself.) The actual elevation of the nerve head is 1 mm. for every 3 diopters (3D) of choking.

Primary Optic Atrophy.—This condition occurs as a result of direct pressure upon the optic nerve from solid tumors, cysts, trauma, or from inflammatory, degenerative or toxic lesions, primarily or secondarily involving the optic pathways.

A progressive reduction in visual acuity occurs. Usually, the fields become constricted concentrically, unless there is pressure upon the optic chiasm from a pituitary lesion. Then the fields take the form of bitemporal hemianopsia. If the tumor extends just posterior to the optic chiasm, thereby involving the optic tract, then the field defect takes the form of homonymous hemianopsia.

Ophthalmoscopic examination shows the disc to be white or bluish white; its margins are sharply defined and regular; the physiological cupping is often exaggerated, and the lamina cribrosa is plainly seen; the small vessels over the disc disappear, and the larger vessels are usually diminished in caliber. When the atrophy is advanced the disc has the appearance of a full moon in a cloudless sky.

There are many complicated theoretical considerations attending the technique of ophthalmoscopic study which, for the sake of simplicity, are omitted here. If the reader will follow the above instructions, he will, with practice, become proficient in the art of ophthalmoscopic diagnosis as applied to neurology.

3. OCULOMOTOR ⎫
4. TROCHLEAR ⎬ Motor
6. ABDUCENS ⎭

These nerves form a functional unit in that they are all concerned with movement of the extrinsic and intrinsic eye muscles. For convenience sake, they are grouped together in the examination.

ANATOMY. **Oculomotor Nerve.**—This nerve supplies all of the extrinsic muscles of the eye (including the levator palpebrae superioris) except the lateral rectus and superior oblique. It also supplies, through its connections with the ciliary ganglion, the constrictor muscle of the pupil and the ciliary muscles.

The fibers of the oculomotor nerve arise from a nucleus in the midbrain just ventral to the anterior end of the cerebral aqueduct (Fig. 10).

On emerging from the brain, the nerve passes between the superior cerebellar and the posterior cerebral arteries, and then pierces the dura mater in front of and lateral to the posterior clinoid process. It runs along the lateral wall of the cavernous sinus and divides into two branches which enter the orbit through the superior orbital fissure.

Trochlear Nerve.—This nerve, the smallest of the cranial nerves, supplies only the superior oblique muscle of the eyeball. Its nucleus lies just below the oculomotor nucleus (Fig. 10). It is unique in that it decussates with its fellow of the opposite side in the anterior medullary velum and emerges just behind the inferior colliculus. It then passes directly across the cerebellar peduncle and winds forward around the cerebral peduncle just above the pons. It pierces the dura just behind the posterior clinoid process and passes forward in the wall of the cavernous sinus, entering the orbit through the superior orbital fissure.

Abducens Nerve.—This nerve supplies the lateral rectus muscle of the eyeball. Its nucleus lies in the dorsal portion of the pons just posterior to the facial nucleus. Its fibers leave the nucleus on its dorsal and medial surfaces, pass through the pons, and emerge between the lower border of the pons and the upper end of the medulla oblongata (Fig. 10). It pierces the dura mater at the dorsum sellae of the sphenoid, runs through the

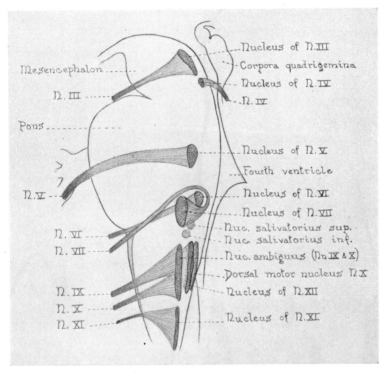

FIG. 10. Diagram of the motor nuclei of the cranial nerves.
(Modified from Ranson)

notch in the bone below the posterior clinoid process, and passes forward through the cavernous sinus, lateral to the internal carotid artery.

The nuclei of the third, fourth and sixth cranial nerves have connections and ramifications which are derived from many sources. Not only are the three nuclei themselves intimately connected, but they receive connections from other cranial nerves, chiefly, the optic, trigeminal, auditory and vestibular, and the voluntary motor pathways. These various connections provide for voluntary movements of the eyeballs, for reflex ocular movements, and for accommodation in response to vestibular, visual and auditory stimuli.

CLINICAL.—Ordinarily, the only subjective finding elicited when there is involvement of the third, fourth and sixth nerves is diplopia (double vision). The patient complains either of blurred vision, or actual double vision when focusing in certain directions. A lead as to the muscle involved is often obtained by asking whether the double vision occurs when looking to the right, left, upward, or downward. In extra-ocular palsies of long standing, the patient sometimes learns to suppress the image derived from one eye, and double vision will then cease to occur.

In testing for extra-ocular muscle weakness, the patient is asked to look at the finger tip of the examiner, following the movements of the finger with the eyes without moving the head. The finger is moved to the right, left, upward and downward. It is often difficult to identify a squint by inspection alone

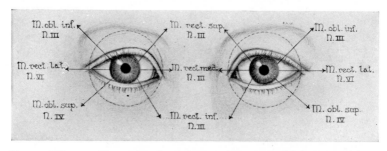

FIG. 11. Diagram illustrating the action of the external muscles of the eyes.

unless there is fairly well marked weakness, so the patient is asked to indicate when he sees the finger doubly. The weakened muscle may be identified easily in this manner (Fig. 11).

The same test is used when searching for nystagmus. This phenomenon is an important localizing sign in neurology. Ordinarily, it does not make its appearance when the eyes remain in the position which they assume spontaneously, but only when the eyes are deviated from this position. The characteristic movements of the eyes when true nystagmus is present are as follows: There is a quick phase (jerk) in the direction of the voluntary movement of the eyes, followed by a slow phase in which the eyes return to their position of rest. Both eyes move in unison. This sequence is repeated over and over again as long as the patient continues to look away from the position of rest. Nystagmus usually takes place in a horizontal plane, but certain rotary movements are often discernible—clockwise rotation on movement of the eyes to the left, and counter-clockwise when turned to the right. Nystagmus in a vertical plane is seldom seen.

Great care is necessary in using the term "nystagmus," as the novice often finds nystagmus in almost every patient he examines. The term should be used only when the two phases (quick jerk in the direction of voluntary movement, followed by a slow return to the position of rest) are present, and when the movements are well sustained. Nystagmoid jerks often occur in tired or nervous patients when trying to fix on an object to the right or left, which requires extreme deviation of the eyes.

Patients with severe visual defects from any cause often present constantly sustained horizontal or vertical nystagmus. The completely blind may have nystagmus but this must not be confused with the "searching movements" so often present.

The essential component of nystagmus is the slow phase, which implies a failure of the eyes to maintain a position to which they are voluntarily moved (quick phase). It may be regarded, therefore, as a deficiency of tonus in the muscles which maintain postures of the eyes, i.e., a form of hypotonia.

Nystagmus occurs in a variety of organic diseases of the nervous system involving the midbrain, pons, cerebellum, vestibular pathways, and the cervical cord. It is especially characteristic in cerebellar disease and disorders of the vestibular apparatus.

Ptosis (drooping of the upper eyelid) results from paralysis of the levator palpebrae superioris muscle which is supplied by the third cranial nerve. Usually, ptosis is associated with complete paralysis of all the other muscles supplied by the third nerve, including the constrictor of the iris and the ciliary muscle. In these circumstances, there is inability to move the eye upward, directly downward, or directly inward, although a slight downward and outward movement can be executed by the superior oblique. The pupil is dilated due to paralysis of the constrictor muscle of the iris, and does not contract either to light or accommodation. Complete third nerve paralysis is most frequently of syphilitic origin but is not uncommon in aneurism of the Circle of Willis. Incomplete paralysis, affecting one or more muscles supplied by the third nerve, is more frequently seen than complete paralysis. Trauma and tumors in the region of the sella turcica are perhaps the most important acquired causes of incomplete third nerve paralysis.

Paralysis of the sixth nerve is the most common of the extra-ocular palsies. Only the lateral rectus muscle is involved (Fig. 11). Consequently, there is double vision on looking laterally to the involved side. In old cases, in which contracture of the non-paralyzed internal rectus has occurred, an internal strabismus results (cross-eye). Due to the relatively long course of this nerve, it is particularly liable to injury from trauma, tumors, abscess, or general increased intracranial pressure from any cause. Therefore, its involvement has only a limited value as a focal sign in diagnosis.

Conjugate movements.—It is interesting that movements of individual eye muscles have no representation in the motor cortex or its projection system. However, conjugate movements are well represented, especially conjugate movements to one side which are often accompanied also by turning the head in the same direction. When the cortex discharges, the eyes are conjugately directed toward the opposite side. In the paralytic period after a convulsion, or from a destructive cortical lesion, the conjugate deviation is toward the side affected. Eye movements are probably never long affected by involvement of one cerebral hemisphere alone, because, as in closure of the eye-lids, there is bilateral cortical representation.

There is an intricate coördinating center (or centers) be-tween the cortical neurons and the nuclei of the separate extra-ocular muscles, located in the midbrain. Lesions in this area may cause dissociation of eye movements or total external oph-thalmoplegia.

Before leaving the examination of extra-ocular movements, a word should be said with regard to the palpebral fissures. Narrowing of the palpebral fissure (pseudoptosis) occurs as a result of destructive lesions of the cervical sympathetic trunk. The levator palpebrae has a dual innervation, the chief supply coming from the oculomotor fibers, but there is an involuntary component from the cervical sympathetics. The cervical sympa-thetic syndrome (Horner's syndrome) consists of the following findings on the side where the sympathetic trunk is affected:

1. Narrowing of palpebral fissure (pseudoptosis).
2. Enophthalmos.
3. Contraction of the pupil due to paralysis of the dilator mechanism of the iris.
4. Absence of sweating over the face and neck.
5. Vasodilatation of the vessels of the head and neck.

A careful examination of the pupils often yields important information relative to organic disorders of the nervous system. The size of the pupils should first be noted in bright and dim light. Are they equal in size? Are they regular in outline? Do they respond promptly to light and accommodation? Do they react to pain (ciliospinal reflex)?

In testing for the reaction of the pupil to light, the patient looks at the most distant corner of the examining room. An electric light (the ophthalmoscopic light is usually strong enough) is then held out of the line of vision several inches from the eye to be tested. As the light is flashed on and off, the response of the pupil is observed. The light should not be placed in the line of vision, because the response of the pupil may be an accommodation reflex instead of a light reflex.

The accommodation reflex is elicited by having the patient

alternately look at some distant object and a near object and noting the corresponding change in the size of the pupil.

The ciliospinal reflex is obtained by pinching the skin of the patient's neck. The slight pain produced causes the pupil to dilate momentarily. This reflex is difficult to obtain in a brightly lighted room. This test is important in lesions involving the cervical sympathetic trunk. It is also useful in obtaining transient dilatation of the pupil for ophthalmoscopic examinations (p. 26).

5. The Trigeminal (*sensory and motor*)

ANATOMY.—The trigeminal nerve is the largest of the cranial nerves. The great sensory portion supplies the face and head, and the smaller motor portion supplies the muscles of mastication.

Sensory Portion.—The sensory root of the fifth nerve has its origin in the gasserian semilunar ganglion. The cells of this ganglion are unipolar like those of the spinal ganglia. The fibers of these cells bifurcate; the external branches pass outward and form the peripheral sensory root; the internal branches pass into the substance of the pons, and there give off ascending and descending branches. The ascending branches pass to a terminal nucleus in the pons beneath the floor of the fourth ventricle, the main sensory nucleus of the trigeminus (Fig. 12). The descending branches pass downward in the pons and medulla, as far as the cervical portion of the spinal cord, and form the spinal tract of the trigeminal nerve and end in the nucleus of the spinal tract of the trigeminus. The nucleus of the spinal tract relays sensations of pain and temperature while the main sensory nucleus relays touch sensations. This distinction is important clinically because the spinal tract of the trigeminus may be interrupted thus abolishing pain and temperature sense on the same side of the face without disturbing touch sensibility. Thus, the nuclei of the trigeminus reach the whole length of the pons and medulla. Its cortical center is in the lower part of the postcentral convolution.

The gasserian ganglion (semilunar ganglion) occupies a cavity in the dura mater near the apex of the petrous portion of the

temporal bone known as Meckel's cave—a diverticulum of
the subarachnoid space. The ganglion receives on its medial
portion filaments from the carotid plexus of the sympathetic

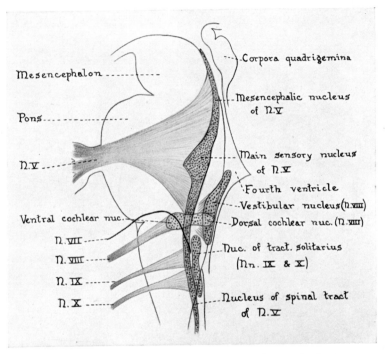

FIG. 12. Diagram of the sensory nuclei of the human brain-stem.
(Modified from Ranson)

system. It gives off in the middle fossa of the skull small
branches to the dura mater, the tentorium, and the falx cerebri.
Three large nerves emerge from its anterior margin: 1. Ophthalmic. 2. Maxillary. 3. Mandibular. These three branches are
usually referred to as the first, second and third divisions of the
fifth nerve (Fig. 13).

The first division passes through the superior orbital fissure
into the orbit. It conducts afferent impulses from the eyeball,
the conjunctiva, the skin of the forehead and scalp up to the
vertex, and the mucous membrane of the upper part of the
nasal cavity.

The second division passes through the skull at the foramen

rotundum. In the sphenomaxillary fossa, it is connected with the sphenopalatine ganglion (Meckel's ganglion). It conducts sensory impulses from the upper lip, nose and adjacent part of the cheek, the lower eyelid, the upper teeth and jaw, hard palate, uvula, tonsil, nasopharynx, middle ear and lower part of the nasal cavity.

The third division leaves the skull through the foramen

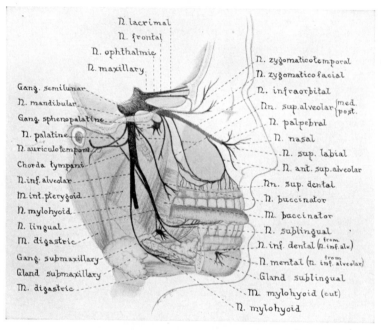

FIG. 13. Distribution of the 2nd and 3rd divisions of the fifth cranial nerve.

ovale; with it runs the motor branch to the muscles of mastication. It conducts sensory impulses from the lower part of the face, the posterior part of the temple, the anterior part of the external auditory meatus, the pinna of the ear, the lower lip, also the lower teeth and gums, the tongue, floor of the mouth, inner side of the cheek and salivary glands.

Motor Portion.—The motor nucleus of the trigeminus lies deeply in the substance of the pons (Fig. 10). The fibers, which take their origin here, form the motor root and run with the mandibular (third division) nerve to supply the muscles of mastication, masseters, temporals and pterygoids.

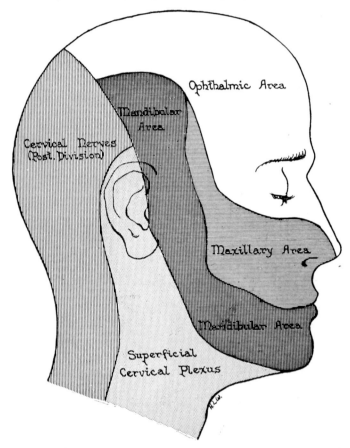

Fig. 14. Diagram showing the superficial sensory distribution of the trigeminal nerve.

CLINICAL.—In testing sensation in the fifth nerve distribution, it is necessary to have a clear mental picture of the exact cutaneous areas supplied by this nerve (Fig. 14). The following types of sensation are tested for: 1. Pain and temperature. 2. Light touch. Deep pressure and muscle sense are conducted through the facial nerve.

In testing for pain, an ordinary straight pin pushed through the end of a tongue depressor is a simple, satisfactory instrument. In estimating the amount of pressure necessary to produce a distinctly painful sensation from the pin prick, the examiner should try the test first on his own face. Nearly identical spots on each side of the face should be tested alternately, the patient indicating any difference in the amount of pain produced. Should one side seem to be less painful than the other, it is well to repeat the test and deliberately use more pressure on the suspected side. If the second test yields the same results as the first, a true reduction in pain sensibility may be recorded. The three divisional distributions of each nerve should be tested separately, as it is not uncommon to have but one division involved.

Variations in temperature sense are tested by means of test tubes filled with hot and cold water (see section on spinal cord examination).

In testing for variations in the sense of light touch, a small piece of absorbent cotton attached to a wooden applicator is used. The examination is confined to those parts relatively free of hair. With the eyes closed, the patient is asked to identify each touch or stroke of the cotton. A very satisfactory gross examination of touch sensibility may be obtained by gently stroking either side of the face with the finger tips. If there is any degree of sensory loss present, it usually will be recognized by this test alone.

The corneal reflex is the most delicate and accurate test of sensory disorders of the first division. With the patient looking upward and away from the side being examined, the margin of the cornea is touched with a tiny piece of absorbent cotton. If normal sensibility is present, the eyelids will be closed promptly. If there is a diminution of sensibility, the cornea may be stroked without blinking of the lids. The conjunctival reflex is tested in the same manner, touching the conjunctiva instead of the cornea. However, the conjunctiva is much less sensitive than the cornea and this test is less delicate than the true corneal reflex.

The motor portion of the fifth nerve is readily tested by palpating the masseter and temporal muscles when the patient clinches his teeth. In unilateral paralysis of the motor fifth nerve there is deviation of the jaw toward the paralyzed side due to failure of the pterygoid muscles to pull the condyloid process forward out of the glenoid fossa.

Destructive lesions of the fifth nerve are most frequently seen in lesions involving the cerebellum, pons and cerebellopontile angle. A tumor or abscess in the posterior fossa of the skull (below the tentorium cerebelli) may cause involvement of the fifth nerve by pressure from the mass. Tumors of the eighth cranial nerve (acoustic neurinomas) are almost always associated with some degree of sensory loss in the distribution of the trigeminus.

Irritative lesions of the nerve or ganglion are far more common. Trigeminal neuralgia (tic douloureux) is one of the most common surgical affections of the nervous system.

7. THE FACIAL (*motor and sensory*)

ANATOMY.—The motor portion of the seventh nerve has its cells of origin in a single nucleus deeply situated in the lower part of the pons (Fig. 10). The facial fibers wind a circuitous course in pontine substance, at one point almost completely encircling the nucleus of the sixth nerve. The nerve leaves the pons at its lower border, just above its junction with the medulla oblongata. It then runs upward and forward to the internal auditory meatus, where it enters the facial canal (fallopian aqueduct). After leaving the pons, the facial and acoustic nerves are intimately associated, the former lying in a groove of the latter. They have a sheath in common formed by continuations of the pia-arachnoid. The nerve leaves the skull at the stylomastoid foramen and supplies all the muscles of the face, the stylohyoid, posterior belly of the digastric, the buccinator, and the platysma. After leaving the stylomastoid foramen, it enters the substance of the parotid gland and breaks up into two main branches, the upper branch supplying the temporal, molar, and infra-orbital regions, and the lower branch supplying the buccal, mandibular and cervical regions.

The sensory root arises from the geniculate ganglion and becomes a part of the seventh nerve in the facial canal. The cells are unipolar, and the single process divides in a T-shaped manner into central and peripheral branches. The central branches form a trunk (intermediate nerve or nerve of Wrisberg), which leaves the facial nerve at the internal auditory meatus. It runs between the facial and acoustic nerves to its entrance in the brain at the lower border of the pons. The fibers of the sensory root pass into the substance of the medulla and end in the upper part of the nucleus of the tractus solitarius. Some of the peripheral branches leave the geniculate ganglion, forming the superficial petrosal nerve, while others continue with the main trunk, leaving it just before it enters the stylomastoid foramen, as the chorda tympani nerve. This sensory portion of the nerve receives sensory impulses from the taste buds on the anterior two-thirds of the tongue. Also, the autonomic fibers, which stimulate the secretion of saliva and tears, run with the facial nerve from the level of the geniculate ganglion outward.

The cortical center of the facial nerve is in the lower part of the precentral convolution. The branches of the facial, which supply the muscles of the upper part of the face, have a cortical connection from each hemisphere (bilateral innervation). The lower branches have a cortical center only in the contralateral hemispheres. These fibers from the cortex pass downward through the internal capsule and decussate before reaching the facial nucleus. Thus, a lesion involving the cortical center of the face, or the pathways from this center to the nucleus, will cause involvement only of the lower part of the face on the contralateral side (supranuclear type of facial paralysis). A lesion involving the nucleus, or the nerve peripheral to the nucleus, will affect all the muscles of the face, often the sensory functions of the nerve as well (peripheral type of facial paralysis).

CLINICAL.—The facial nerve is more frequently involved by diseases of the nervous system than any other nerve, cranial or spinal.

Motor.—Inspection of the patient's face during the history taking is the most satisfactory means of discovering facial nerve palsy of slight degree. Does the patient's face have a one-sided appearance? Does he appear to talk out of one side of his mouth? Does one side seem smoother and freer of wrinkles than the other? When the eyes blink, does one lid fail to close or lag? If weakness of one side appears to be present, does it disappear during emotional stress? Observations such as the above are made in an apparent casual manner and often furnish a clue to facial nerve involvement, when tests of voluntary movements fail.

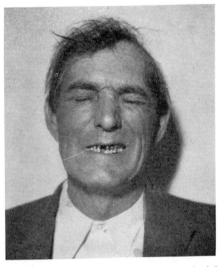

FIG. 15. Supranuclear type of facial weakness in a case of left frontal lobe tumor.

Further information is obtained by asking the patient to show his teeth, whistle, or smile. If the lower branches of the nerve are involved, a distinct asymmetry of the mouth will appear, the lips being drawn further to the sound side. If the same patient laughs at a joke, the asymmetry may completely disappear. During moments of rest, the face at first may appear symmetrical, but on closer examination, the nasolabial fold on the involved side will be found to be "ironed out" or completely absent.

The upper portion of the face is examined by having the patient raise his eyebrows, frown, and shut his eyes tightly. Weakness of the orbicularis oculi may be demonstrated by the examiner trying to open the eyelids against the patient's effort to keep them closed.

The point of distinction between peripheral and supranuclear types of facial paralysis must be stressed because of its importance in neurological diagnosis. In cortical or subcortical lesions involving the facial nerve connections, only the muscles of the lower part of the face (below the lower eyelid) are involved. The explanation of this phenomenon is that the lower

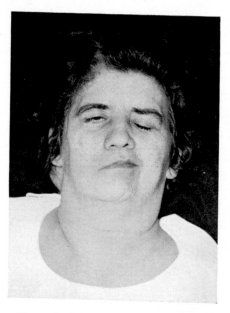

FIG. 16. Infranuclear facial paralysis. Note asymmetry of the mouth and inability to close the eyelids on the affected side.

branches of the nerve have connections with but a single cortical center, and that is in the opposite hemisphere, the upper branches having bilateral cortical connections which keep the muscles of the upper part of the face working when the contralateral cortical connections are out of order (Fig. 15). In the peripheral types of facial paralysis, all the muscles of the face are more or less equally involved, i.e., there is asymmetry when wrinkling the forehead, closing the eyes, or showing the teeth. Paralysis of this sort occurs with destructive lesions anywhere in the course of the nerve from its nucleus in the pons to its peripheral distribution (Fig. 16).

Supranuclear facial weakness occurs in tumors, abscesses, and traumatic lesions involving the frontal, temporal, or parietal lobes of the cerebrum, in capsular hemorrhages (apoplexy), in occlusion of the middle cerebral artery, and a variety of other destructive lesions of the cerebral hemisphere. Peripheral facial palsies occur only in diseases involving the contents of the posterior fossa (cerebellum, pons, cerebellopontile angles, or medulla), or of the facial nerve itself during its course through the bony canal of the skull or after its exit from the stylomastoid foramen.

Hyperacusis is a painful sensitiveness to loud sounds, caused by paralysis of the nerve which supplies the stapedius muscle of the middle ear. It occurs when there is a destructive lesion involving the facial nerve central to the exit of the nerve to the stapedius.

Sensory.—Loss of taste on the anterior two-thirds of the tongue occurs when there is a lesion of the nerve central to the exit of the chorda tympani branch and peripheral to the geniculate ganglion. In nuclear lesions of the facial nerve, loss of taste does not occur. The examination of taste is carried out in the following manner: The patient is asked to put out his tongue and keep it out during the test. A little salt, powdered sugar, or quinine is placed on the tongue and gently rubbed in with a piece of gauze. He then indicates the sensation produced by pointing to the words "salt," "sweet," or "bitter," which are held before him on a chart. Each half of the tongue is tested separately. If the patient puts the tongue back into his mouth, the test is spoiled, as taste buds on the posterior part of the tongue (supplied by the glossopharyngeal) may be stimulated.

A more accurate method is to use a copper wire electrode connected with a weak galvanic current. When the current is applied to the tongue, a peculiar bitter taste is produced.

8. The Acoustic (*sensory*)

The eighth nerve is made up of two sets of fibers which have entirely dissimilar functions: The cochlear (sense of hearing) and the vestibular (sense of balance).

Anatomy. **Cochlear Division.**—This nerve arises from bipolar cells in the spiral ganglion of the cochlea, situated in the petrous portion of the temporal bone. The peripheral fibers pass to the organ of Corti, while the central fibers are directed toward the brain in the cochlear nerve. The nerve passes along the internal auditory meatus with the vestibular and facial nerves, across the subarachnoid space, to enter the cochlear nucleus in the upper part of the medulla (Fig. 12). The supranuclear connections of the cochlear nucleus present an intricate arrangement, the details of which are omitted here for the sake of simplicity. It is sufficient for our purpose to know that each nucleus has a bilateral cortical center located in the superior and transverse temporal gyri. Therefore, a destructive lesion of one temporal lobe does not produce deafness, due to the double cortical representation.

Vestibular Portion.—The vestibular root, the nerve of equilibrium, arises from bipolar cells in the vestibular ganglion situated in the internal auditory meatus. The peripheral fibers end in the vestibular portion of the labyrinth. The central fibers, which collectively form the vestibular nerve, follow the same course as the cochlear nerve into the brain substance. After entering the brain, the fibers divide into ascending and descending branches which terminate in the large vestibular nucleus,

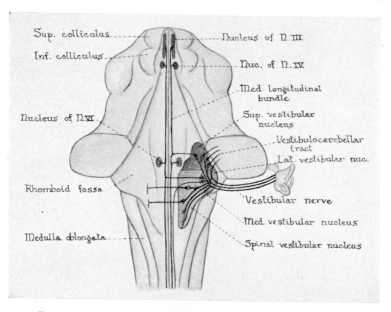

FIG. 17. Diagram of the vestibular nerve, its nuclei and central connections. (Modified from Ranson)

forming an eminence on the floor of the fourth ventricle (Fig. 12). This nucleus has four main divisions:

1. Medial or principal nucleus.
2. Lateral or Deiters' nucleus.

3. Descending or spinal nucleus.

4. Superior nucleus.

The arrangement of these nuclei and some of their connections are shown in Fig. 17.

Some of the connections are for reflex purposes in the brain-stem itself; there are connections with the vestibulo-spinal tract for movements of the trunk and limbs in response to stimulation of the semicircular canals; there are connections with the medial longitudinal bundle, by which fibers descend to the spinal cord and ascend to the midbrain; there are many connections with the cerebellum, the chief ones passing from the superior and lateral (Deiters') nuclei as the vestibulo-cerebellar tract. (See section on the cerebellum.) It will be noticed that there are no important connections with the thalamus and cerebral cortex, for the equilibratory reactions from the semicircular canals are normally performed subconsciously.

The connections with the nuclei of the motor nerves of the eye are made through the medial longitudinal bundle, thus providing for reflex conjugate eye movements which enable one to keep the gaze fixed upon a stationary object while the head is moving.

Within the semicircular canals, a part of the internal ear, are highly specialized end-organs, the function of which is concerned chiefly with the maintenance of bodily equilibrium. The three canals lie approximately at right angles to each other. Each one is dilated at one end to form the ampulla, within which is a patch of sensory epithelium from which hairs project. A movement of the head in any direction causes stimulation of the sensory cells of the vestibular organs. Impulses resulting from these stimuli are transmitted to the vestibular centers in the brain, where they are sorted and analyzed so that an appropriate reaction may be initiated in various parts of the nervous system to compensate for this movement.

CLINICAL.—Disorders of the acoustic nerve commonly accompany surgical lesions of the brain; therefore, it is important that the neurologist have an accurate working knowledge of the simpler diagnostic tests used in otology.

Cochlear.—The chief symptoms referable to the cochlear division of the acoustic nerve are deafness and tinnitus.

Hearing may be satisfactorily tested by determining the distance from each ear that the tick of an ordinary watch can be heard. Any difference between the two sides is of more importance to the neurologist than the absolute value of auditory acuity. A more exact test is made by the use of tuning forks. A single medium pitched fork ($C' = 256$ vibrations per second is to be preferred) is sufficient equipment to detect a degree of deafness having significance in diagnostic neurology. The Rinne test is performed in the following manner: The fork is set vibrating by striking it against the hand. The end of the fork is held snugly against the tip of the mastoid process, and the patient indicates when he ceases to hear the musical note (bone conduction). The position of the fork is changed, so that the prongs are close to the external auditory meatus. The patient again indicates when the note is no longer heard (air conduction). Normally, the musical note is heard by air conduction approximately twice as long as by bone conduction. In deafness due to disease of the labyrinth or the cochlear nerve, the normal relationship is maintained, but the duration of each is decreased. In middle ear disease, or blocking of the external auditory canal by wax, the relationship between air and bone conduction is reversed, the hearing by bone conduction being greater than by air conduction.

The Weber test is performed by placing the end of the vibrating fork on the vertex of the head, exactly in the midline. The patient indicates in which ear the musical note is heard better. Normally, it will be heard equally well in both ears. In middle ear disease, or plugging of the external auditory canal, it will be heard better on the affected side. In nerve deafness, the note will be heard better on the sound side. In other words, if the fork is lateralized by this test, some impairment of hearing exists. It is then necessary to consult the results of the Rinne test to determine whether the deafness is due to middle ear disease or nerve deafness. Thus, the two tests afford a check upon each other.

An otoscopic examination should be performed in every case where there is disturbance of hearing. Accumulation of wax in the external auditory canal and inflammatory lesions of the middle ear are by far the most common causes of deafness and tinnitus. The novice can, with a few hours' practice, acquire sufficient skill with the otoscope to recognize gross abnormalities of the auditory canal and ear drum.

Noises in the ear (tinnitus) signify irritation of some part of the auditory apparatus. When it is due to intracranial disease, it is usually accompanied by some degree of deafness. It may be caused, also, by wax on the drum, middle ear disorders, prolonged exposure to loud noises and quinine poisoning. When it occurs in a patient with a neurological disorder, this symptom may have a significance of great importance. In tumors of the eighth nerve (acoustic neurinomas), tinnitus is usually the first symptom to make its appearance. In labyrinthian disturbances (Ménière's disease), it is often the most aggravating complaint. In aneurisms or hemangiomas of the brain, it may be the only subjective finding.

Noises in the ear may be described by the patient in a varied manner. Some say the sounds resemble "a metal hammer pounding on an anvil," or "ticking of a clock," or "beating of a drum," or "the swish of rushing water." In any event, tinnitus is a most distressing symptom, since it not only annoys the patient by day but often prevents sleep at night.

Vestibular Portion.—Ordinarily, when there is a disturbance of the vestibular nerve, the only symptoms are dizziness (vertigo) and unsteadiness of gait. Since the vestibular apparatus is so closely bound up with the cerebellum in function, a detailed discussion of the findings in disorders of the vestibulocerebellar apparatus will be given under the section dealing with cerebellar symptomatology.

When the vestibular apparatus (semicircular canals and vestibular nerve or its nuclei) is irritated, dizziness, nystagmus, incoördination and often nausea are produced.

By use of the Bárány test, we are able to determine whether the nerve with its end-organs and nuclear connections is intact.

The test in all its details is quite elaborate and too complex for use in the routine neurological examination. However, one part, the caloric test, is easy to perform and yields sufficient information regarding the integrity of the nerve to justify its use in every case suspected of having vestibular involvement.

The Caloric Test of Bárány.—Before the caloric test is started, the patient should be instructed in the tests for incoördination and nystagmus. He should indicate promptly the onset of dizziness or nausea.

The test is performed with the patient sitting upright in a chair or bed. The ear on the suspected side is examined first. An ordinary bulb syringe, a pitcher of cold water (18°C to 20°C), a kidney shaped basin, and two towels are all the equipment needed. The external auditory canal is irrigated slowly, care being taken not to direct the stream of water directly upon the ear-drum. After 100 c.c. of water have been used, the external ear is dried, and the following observations are made:

1. Nystagmus, the type and direction.
2. Past-pointing tests with each hand (see section on cerebellum).
3. Time elapsing before onset of dizziness or nausea.

Then the position of the head is changed by bending it forward on the chest. Any change in the direction of nystagmus in this position is noted. Then the head is changed back to its original position, and the same observations repeated. After the change of position, the reaction is usually intensified.

If the right ear has been irrigated, the normal response to this test, performed in the manner just indicated, will be:

1. Onset of dizziness within 2 minutes after the irrigation is started.
2. Lateral and rotary nystagmus to the left.
3. Past-pointing, more marked on the right side.
4. Sense of nausea usually develops and may be followed by vomiting at the height of the vertigo.
5. When the head is flexed on the chest, the nystagmus may become more pronounced to the right side.

6. Changing the head back to the original position usually exaggerates the dizziness, nystagmus and past-pointing.

If there is complete blocking of the nerve and the labyrinth is "dead," there will be no nystagmus, vertigo, or past-pointing. If there is no nystagmus, but the other reactions are present, it may be inferred that the connections of the nerve with the median longitudinal bundle, through which the extra-ocular muscles are innervated, are affected.

If there is an incomplete blocking of the nerve or its connections, the whole response will be delayed or reduced in intensity.

If the response to this test is absent or decreased, it indicates a destructive lesion in the labyrinth or the posterior fossa of the skull, cerebellum, pons, medulla or cerebellopontile angle. The response is often highly exaggerated in supratentorial tumors.

9. THE GLOSSOPHARYNGEAL (*motor and sensory*)

ANATOMY.—As its name implies, the branches of this nerve are distributed to the tongue and pharynx. The sensory branches supply ordinary sensation to the mucous membrane of the pharynx, palatine tonsils and fauces, and the sense of taste to the posterior one-third of the tongue. Its motor fibers partially supply the constrictor muscles of the pharynx, and wholly supply the stylopharyngeus muscles. Loss of motor function does not affect swallowing or other pharyngeal movements significantly.

The motor fibers arise from a nucleus in the medulla (nucleus ambiguus), which is common to the glossopharyngeal, vagus and accessory nerves (Fig. 10).

The sensory fibers arise from two small ganglia situated on the trunk of the nerve where it leaves the skull at the jugular foramen. The central branches end in the nucleus of tractus solitarius in the medulla, and the peripheral branches form the sensory nerve for the pharynx, tonsils and posterior one-third of the tongue.

The glossopharyngeal nerve leaves the skull through the jugular foramen, lateral to, and in front of the vagus and accessory nerves. It then passes forward between the internal jugular vein and the internal carotid artery, and descends in the neck in front of the artery beneath the styloid process to the lower border of the stylopharyngeus muscle. Then, it curves forward under the hypoglossal nerve and is distributed to the palatine tonsil and the mucous membrane of the pharynx and base of the tongue.

CLINICAL.—Loss of function of the glossopharyngeal nerve causes anesthesia of the back of the tongue, tonsil and pharynx, and loss of taste on the posterior one-third of the tongue.

Loss of sensation is best demonstrated by touching the posterior wall of the pharynx or the pharyngeal tonsil with a wooden tongue depressor. If there is a prompt contraction of the pharyngeal muscles, with or without gagging, the integrity of the nerve may be assumed to be intact (pharyngeal reflex).

Testing for taste on the posterior one-third of the tongue is difficult unless one is provided with a long copper electrode and a galvanic cell. This test is usually of academic interest only in the neurological examination.

Irritative lesions of the ninth nerve are occasionally encountered. Glossopharyngeal neuralgia (tic douloureux) is a painful malady limited to the sensory distribution of the nerve, and has the identical characteristics, except for the difference in distribution, of trigeminal neuralgia.

10. THE VAGUS (*motor and sensory*)

ANATOMY.—The tenth nerve has the most extensive course and distribution of any of the cranial nerves. It belongs chiefly to the autonomic nervous system (parasympathetic), although it does supply fibers to skeletal muscles and a limited amount of skin.

The motor fibers arise from two nuclei: 1. Nucleus ambiguus. 2. Dorsal motor nucleus of the vagus.

The motor fibers arising from the nucleus ambiguus supply the larynx, soft palate and part of the pharynx. The fibers arising from the dorsal motor nucleus of the vagus are purely autonomic fibers and carry the efferent impulses to the thoracic and abdominal viscera.

The sensory fibers arise from two ganglia (jugular and nodosum) that lie on the root of the nerve at the level of the jugular foramen where the nerve leaves the skull. The central fibers enter the medulla, and most of them end in the nucleus of the tractus solitarius. This portion of the nerve conducts sensory impulses from the pharynx, larynx, trachea, esophagus and the thoracic and abdominal viscera. The sensory fibers, supplying the skin of the external ear, probably end in the nucleus of the spinal tract of the trigeminus.

CLINICAL.—The neurological signs arising from vagal disorders are few in number as compared with the great complexity of function centered in this nerve. The symptoms of vagus involvement vary with the site and extent of the lesion. If the whole trunk is affected, there is unilateral paralysis of the palate, pharynx, and larynx, together with anesthesia of the larynx on the affected side. The symptoms arising from such a unilateral lesion are hoarseness caused by paralysis of the vocal cord, and regurgitation of fluids through the nose due to paralysis of the soft palate. The method of testing for paralysis of the soft palate consists of observing its movements when the patient utters the syllable "ah." Normally, the median raphé rises straight up, but if one side is weak, the raphé deviates to the sound side. Also, observe the patient attempting to swallow water; it is likely he will strangle and regurgitate the water through his nose.

Projectile vomiting (cerebral vomiting) is one of the classic signs of increased intracranial pressure, particularly when the pressure is due to tumors in the posterior fossa of the skull. The mechanism responsible for this type of vomiting is still imperfectly understood, but it is believed by many to be due to irritation of the tractus solitarius, or its nucleus, through which the impulses for ordinary vomiting are relayed from the gastric mucosa. Since the vagus nerve is so intimately associated with this fasciculus and its nucleus, cerebral vomiting, then, may be considered as a vagal phenomenon. In certain tumors arising in the floor of the fourth ventricle, persistent vomiting occurs as the result of direct involvement of the vagal nuclei and may, therefore, be a persistent symptom for weeks or months before the signs of increased intracranial pressure are evident.

The slow pulse, which is commonly observed in increased intracranial pressure, is probably due to irritation of the vagus, since these nerves comprise the inhibitory or slowing mechanism of the heart. Lesions which destroy the function of both vagi naturally will remove this slowing mechanism and allow the heart to "run away" as the result of removing the controls from the accelerator innervation (sympathetic).

11. THE SPINAL ACCESSORY (*motor*)

ANATOMY.—The accessory nerve consists of an intracranial and spinal portion; however, the cerebral portion can properly be considered a part of the vagus. The intracranial branch arises from the dorsal motor nucleus of the vagus and passes through the jugular foramen with the spinal portion and with the ninth and tenth cranial nerves. After leaving the brain-stem, it descends to join the spinal portion. At the jugular foramen, the nerve divides into an internal and external branch, the fibers from the bulb forming the internal branch which soon joins the vagus nerve at the ganglion nodosum and is distributed with it to the muscles of the larynx and pharynx. The external branch is made up wholly of fibers from the spinal portion and is distributed to the sternocleidomastoid muscle and the upper part of the trapezius.

The spinal root takes origin from the anterior gray column of the first five or six segments of the cervical spinal cord. The root ascends beside the spinal cord, passes through the foramen magnum and joins the bulbar portion as described above.

CLINICAL.—The examination for spinal accessory function is made by having the patient turn his head to the right and left, while the examiner feels the contraction of the sternocleidomastoid muscles which are chiefly responsible for these movements. When one muscle is weak, the head cannot be completely turned to the opposite side. In testing for the action of the upper trapezii, have the patient forcibly elevate the shoulders, while the examiner palpates the upper portion of the muscles. If one side is weak, the shoulder will be incompletely raised on the affected side. Also, when the shoulders are viewed from the rear, there will be noted a downward and outward displacement of the scapula on the involved side.

The spinal portion of the accessory nerve differs only in its unusual origin from other motor nerves. The muscles it supplies together with other muscles about the neck and shoulders are often involved in spasmodic torticollis.

12. THE HYPOGLOSSAL (*motor*)

ANATOMY.—The nucleus of the hypoglossal nerve is a cylindrical mass of cells, lying in the inferior part of the medulla in the floor of the fourth ventricle. The fibers leave the medulla at the lateral margin of the pyramid and course along the floor of the skull to the point of exit at the anterior condyloid foramen. After leaving the skull it is joined by branches from the first and second cervical nerves, which soon leave the main trunk, as the descendens hypoglossi, to be distributed to the sternohyoid and sternothyroid muscles. The main trunk of the nerve is distributed to the extrinsic and intrinsic muscles of the tongue.

CLINICAL.—The signs of glossal paralysis are easily demonstrated. When the tongue is protruded, it deviates toward the paralyzed side. This is due to the unopposed action of the geniohyoglossus muscle on the healthy side which, because of the course of its muscle fibers, tends to draw the tongue toward the midline. The paralyzed side of the tongue becomes atrophied and wrinkled. The patient usually complains of difficulty in mastication and articulation, especially when the onset of the paralysis is sudden. After a time, he becomes accustomed to the deformity, and nothing other than a "lisping" speech will be noted. Although a patient learns to compensate well

for unilateral hypoglossal paralysis, bilateral paralysis produces a permanent defect. Since the cortical representation of
the tongue is from the contralateral motor cortex, cerebral
lesions often produce transient paresis of the opposite side of
the tongue.

Slight involvement of the hypoglossal nerve may be demonstrated only by deviation of the tongue from the midline when
fully protruded. Isolated involvement of this nerve from intracranial disease is seldom seen.

CHAPTER III

THE CEREBRUM

The cerebral hemispheres, from the phylogenetic point of view, are the youngest portions of the brain. The stage of development of these structures represents the only essential difference between the brains of humans and lower animals. The higher one ascends in the animal scale, the greater the relative size and development of the cerebral hemispheres. As early as the second century A.D., Galen taught that the cerebrum is the organ of intelligence and conscious sensations. All modern investigation has confirmed his theory.

After it was established that the cerebrum is the organ of higher psychical activities, the question naturally arose whether different parts of the cortex possess functions peculiar to their locations, or whether the cerebrum acts as a unit, functionally equivalent throughout. This question remained unanswered until the latter part of the nineteenth century when the cerebrum, exposed in the living animal, was stimulated electrically. This marked the beginning of all modern views on cerebral localization. The first effect of this work led to an extreme view in which the different motor and sensory areas of the brain were thought to be definitely circumscribed and sharply separated from each other in a mosaic pattern. The centers were plotted for various functions, each sharply separated from the other.

All recent work tends to modify this view. In fact, cortical diagrams, so prevalent in the latter part of the nineteenth century, become dimmer and dimmer until now about the only sharply defined pattern remaining is the projection area of the retina upon the calcarine area of the occipital lobe. Although but little definite localization of centers, in the old sense, is apparent, nevertheless, certain physiological changes have been demonstrated to occur more frequently with lesions at some sites than at others. By analysis of these physiological changes, the clinical neurologist is able to localize the site of lesions of the cerebral hemispheres with reasonable accuracy.

The different parts of the cerebral hemispheres are connected by association tracts, and with lower levels by the great afferent and efferent pathways. Each hemisphere is connected with the other by a broad white band of commissural fibers known as the *corpus callosum*. The fibers of which it is composed arise in various parts of each hemisphere, then cross to

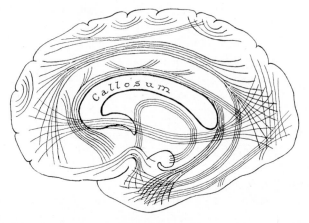

FIG. 18. Diagram showing some of the chief association tracts of the cerebral hemisphere, seen from the medial surface. (After Herrick)

the opposite side where they connect both similar and dissimilar portions of the cortex. Some cortical areas are supplied with these commissural fibers better than others, few, if any, being associated with the visual cortex (Fig. 18).

At the base of each cerebral hemisphere, several nuclear masses are located. From the standpoint of clinical neurology the most important of these are the corpus striatum and the thalamus.

The corpus striatum is composed of the caudate and lenticular nuclei, between which lies the anterior limb of the internal capsule. A discussion of the form and function of the corpus striatum is given at the end of this chapter.

The thalamus is the great sensory nucleus of the brain. It is here that all sensory impulses are received and transmitted to the appropriate centers in the cerebral cortex.

In making a systematic neurological examination, it is convenient to divide the cerebral cortex into its anatomical lobes and consider each separately as though it were a unit, so that we may better localize the cerebral disease which is producing symptoms. By means of the more important fissures or convolutions, the cerebral cortex is marked into well-defined areas

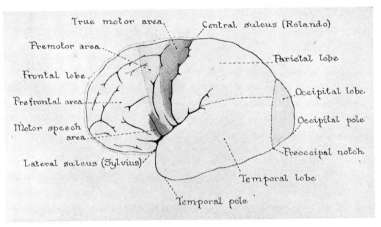

FIG. 19. Lobes of the left cerebral hemisphere (diagrammatic). Areas of known functional activity of the left frontal lobe are indicated.

known as the frontal, parietal, temporal, and occipital lobes (Fig. 19).

A. THE FRONTAL LOBE

ANATOMY AND PHYSIOLOGY.—The frontal lobe comprises the anterior one-third of each cerebral hemisphere in man. The posterior border of the external surface of the lobe is marked by the central fissure (Rolando), and the inferior border by the lateral cerebral fissure (Sylvius). Three principal sulci (fissures) may be identified in the frontal lobe: the precentral, the superior frontal, and the inferior frontal sulci. Between the precentral and central sulci lies the precentral gyrus, the great motor area of the cerebral cortex. The remainder of the frontal lobe is divided into three gyri (convolutions): the superior, middle, and inferior. The middle gyrus is traversed by the ill-defined middle frontal sulcus (Fig. 22).

From the standpoint of functional activity, the frontal lobe may be divided into four well-defined areas. Undoubtedly, there are more, but with the knowledge of frontal lobe activity in its present nebulous state only four need be recognized from the point of view of clinical neurology. These areas are: (1) the prefrontal area; (2) the true motor area; (3) the premotor area; (4) the motor speech area (Fig. 19).

1. **The Prefrontal Area.**—Knowledge of functional activity of the prefrontal area in man is limited to such deductions as can be made from the effect of experimental lesions in lower animals and from the effect of disease upon this area in man.

Fulton and Jacobsen have shown that when *both* prefrontal areas are removed in monkeys, the animals exhibit a great increase in motor activity with constant restlessness. With the increase of motor activity, there is an associated marked increase in appetite, but in spite of this, the animal loses weight. If the premotor and the true motor areas are undamaged, no permanent alterations of posture and no motor defects occur. The "mental" defect produced by such a lesion consists of an apparent "memory" loss of acquired skilled acts, particularly the capacity to perform a series of maneuvers spread out in time. There is some evidence for the belief that the animal has no appreciation of the passage of time.

The effects of disease of the prefrontal areas in man have yielded very discordant results, some reporting no changes, and some very severe alterations of intelligence and character. The consensus of opinion from the observations of recent authors seems to be that disease or injury of the prefrontal area, especially bilateral, produces characteristic changes in the intellectual status of the patient. His power of attention is lessened; there is difficulty in comprehension, especially the acquisition of new material; there may be marked deficiencies and distortions of the emotional life; he may show marked irritability and slowness in the execution of acts or the formation of ideas. All of these psychic symptoms may be present, yet his memory show little impairment.

Some of the confusion with regard to prefrontal activity has arisen from failure to recognize that the frontal lobes are not functionally equivalent. There is an abundance of clinical evidence to show that in right-handed persons, the left frontal lobe is dominant, the reverse being true in the left-handed. Space-occupying lesions limited to the right frontal lobe in the right-handed produce fewer "mental" symptoms than a similarly placed lesion in the left hemisphere. However, amputation of either prefrontal area in man is followed by surprisingly few demonstrable defects in the psychic state. Unilateral prefrontal lobectomy is, therefore, an entirely acceptable procedure when dealing with surgical lesions in the anterior cranial fossa.

Interpretation of the cause of symptoms which are attributed to the prefrontal areas should be made with due respect for the possibility that irritation rather than the destruction of tissues may be the inciting factor. The fact that a large tumor involving the dominant frontal lobe causes certain "mental" symptoms does not necessarily prove that such symptoms arise wholly from destruction of prefrontal tissue. It is a common experience in the neurosurgical clinics to see patients with marked "mental" symptoms regain their higher psychical reactions when a neoplasm is removed from the dominant prefrontal area; even when in the process of removal there has been more extensive destruction of cortical tissue than that produced by the tumor itself. Moreover, the heightened intracranial pressure which occurs with most neoplasms affects not only the local area but the entire content of the cranial cavity. For this reason, the effects of inflammatory, neoplastic and degenerative lesions cannot be taken as final evidence in evaluating normal functional activity.

2. The True Motor Area.—The motor cortex is situated immediately anterior to the central fissure (Rolando) and occupies a large portion of the precentral convolution (Fig. 19). It is wider superiorly than inferiorly; in fact, at the inferior

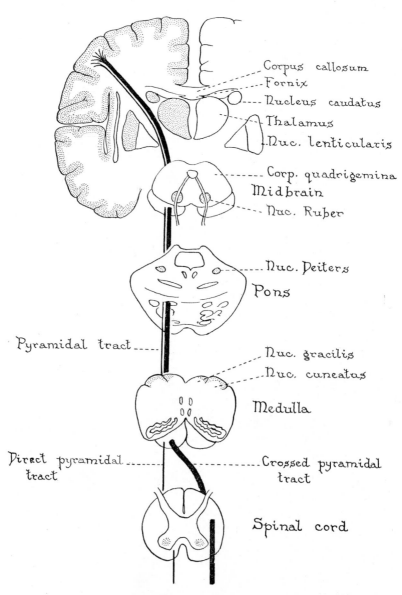

Corpus callosum
Fornix
Nucleus caudatus
Thalamus
Nuc. lenticularis

Corp. quadrigemina
Midbrain
Nuc. Ruber

Nuc. Deiters
Pons

Pyramidal tract

Nuc. gracilis
Nuc. cuneatus

Medulla

Direct pyramidal tract

Crossed pyramidal tract

Spinal cord

FIG. 20. Diagram showing the course of the corticospinal tract.
(Modified from Purves-Stewart)

extremity in the region which represents the hand, the motor cells scarcely emerge from the central fissure.

The giant pyramidal cells of Betz (motor cells) identify this area of the cortex beyond all doubt and furnish an absolute guide to the confines of the motor cortex. These cells give rise to axons which form the pyramidal tracts. The pyramidal tracts traverse the white matter of the brain through the internal capsule, the pons, and the medulla, where most of the fibers decussate. At the point of decussation in the medulla, the greater part of the fibers cross to the opposite side of the spinal cord and continue as the lateral corticospinal tract (crossed pyramidal tract) to the connections at different levels with the anterior horn cells. The smaller group of fibers continues without crossing down the cord in the ventral corticospinal tract (direct pyramidal tract, Fig. 20). Another part of the pyramidal tract, the corticobulbar tract, connects the motor cortex with the motor nuclei of the cranial nerves.

The voluntary motor pathways are formed by two-unit chains, the upper motor neurons and the lower motor neurons. The upper motor neurons conduct impulses from the motor cortex to the motor nuclei of the cranial nerves or to the anterior horn cells in the gray matter of the spinal cord. The lower motor neurons conduct these impulses from the motor nuclei of the cranial nerves and the anterior horn cells to the motor end-organs in the skeletal muscles. Thus, these connections bring the motor cortex into direct communication with the motor cells of the brain-stem and the spinal cord. In consequence, the skeletal musculature is brought under voluntary control.

The motor cortex, as it officiates in dispatching voluntary impulses, is influenced by many adjacent and distant areas of the cerebrum. Each voluntary act is the result of a vast number of impulses converging upon the giant pyramidal cells. These cells, although they serve for the final transmission of impulses for voluntary movement, are activated in this process from other sources and probably play but a small part in the initiation of the voluntary action.

The motor cortex is arranged in an orderly manner so that certain parts control special parts of the body. The cortical pattern is represented in an inverted order, the foot center being at the top and the centers for the eyelids, mouth and larynx being at the bottom of the convolution. The thumb center lies next to those of the cranial nerves. This is reflected clinically in the frequent simultaneous twitching of the thumb, index finger and the face in a jacksonian convulsion (Fig. 21). Experimental destruction of any of these areas causes some degree of paralysis in the corresponding parts.

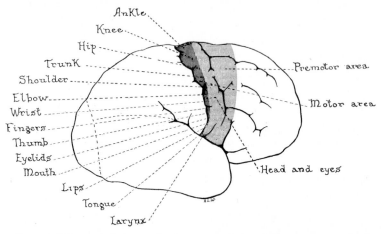

Fig. 21. Diagram of the cerebral motor cortex and the premotor area.

The time-honored conception that a destructive lesion of the motor cortex always produces *paralysis* accompanied by heightened tendon reflexes, spasticity, and finally contractures is certainly open to question in view of recent experimental and clinical data.

When the true motor cortex on one side is removed in a monkey or chimpanzee, the contralateral extremities are at first paralyzed and flaccid. After a few days, the paralysis begins to improve, and at the end of six to eight weeks, the return of function is such that gross movements of the extremities are performed in a nearly normal manner. Most of the permanent residual motor loss consists of clumsiness in finer movements of the fingers and toes. The paralysis is always of the flaccid type and is never associated with spasticity. Tendon reflexes, however, may ultimately become somewhat increased.

If the premotor area is destroyed at the same time, the resulting paralysis is accompanied by heightened tendon reflexes and spasticity. Recovery from a lesion of this type is slower and less complete; in fact, voluntary power in the small muscles of the digits is never regained.

It is evident, therefore, that in the monkey and chimpanzee, destruction of the true motor cortex produces paralysis of the flaccid type, but if the premotor cortex is likewise destroyed, the paralysis is spastic.

Destructive lesions of the motor cortex in man are invariably followed by profound contralateral paralysis. After a period of weeks or months, motor power begins to return, but restoration of function is never comparable to that observed in lower animals. The disturbance is greater in the foot and hand than in the knee or elbow, the hip or shoulder. There is a difference in distribution among the muscle groups of the limbs themselves. In the arm, paralysis is most severe in the extensors, and in the leg, in the flexors. It is difficult to open the hand. The lower limb is rotated outward and the upper limb inward.

In acute lesions, the paralysis is at first flaccid. After a time, the muscles of the paralyzed extremities usually become hypertonic, and the tendon reflexes become exaggerated. As a result of this spasticity, contractures are apt to occur. When the destructive lesion is slow in onset, the flaccid stage is seldom seen, the paralysis being of the spastic variety from the beginning.

What relation the state of spasticity has to the true motor and the premotor areas in man is yet to be shown conclusively. Destructive lesions in man are, as a rule, relatively large, so that it would be most unusual to find one sharply localized to the true motor cortex without some implication of the premotor area. Perhaps this fact explains the occurrence of spasticity in almost all human cases with lesions of the motor cortex. Fulton has seen a case of hemiplegia with a small capsular lesion involving only the middle portion of the internal capsule, in which the affected extremities were completely flaccid over a long period of time. He believes that had the hemorrhage involved the anterior as well as the middle part of the capsule and had thus implicated the projection system both from the motor and the premotor areas, the extremities would have become spastic. Certainly, this observer has demonstrated conclusively on monkeys that spasticity is a product of destruction involving the premotor area, and that lesions limited to the true motor area produce invariably a flaccid paralysis.

However, until more information is accumulated upon the effect of lesions in the true and the premotor cortex in man, we must still cling to the conception that destructive lesions of the motor cortex produce paralysis which, in acute cases, is at first flaccid, and later spastic, and in chronic cases is spastic from the beginning.

3. **The Premotor Area.**—The premotor (psychomotor) area lies immediately in front of the true motor cortex (Fig. 19). Its anterior boundary is not constant, but in general its form resembles closely that of the true motor cortex. The histological structure of the premotor area is similar in every respect to the motor cortex with the exception that the giant pyramidal cells are absent. The strong histological resemblance of these two areas leaves little room for doubt of their close physiological association.

The threshold for electrical excitation of the premotor cortex is higher than that of the motor area, and since excision of this area diminishes voluntary motor control, it probably exerts and directs control over the voluntary musculature.

When the premotor area alone is removed in monkeys, there occurs a transient loss of voluntary motor power in the contralateral extremities with an increased resistance to passive manipulation (spasticity). The tendon reflexes are hyperactive, and the Babinski sign is positive. In addition, involuntary reflex grasping (forced grasping) occurs. After a few days or weeks, all of these phenomena are likely to disappear, but there remains indefinitely a curious reluctance to initiate voluntary movements and an obvious awkwardness in the performance of finely skilled acts.

Opportunity for studying the functional activity of the premotor area in man has been limited because of the rarity of circumscribed lesions confined to this part of the cortex. Such evidence as may be deemed reliable would indicate that the premotor area is the region in which the motion formula for skilled acts is constructed and retained. Development of function in this area apparently results from repeated execution of any skilled performance until a degree of relative perfection in execution is obtained. Handwriting, typewriting, and the playing of musical instruments are good examples of skilled acts, the perfection of which is dependent upon development in the premotor area.

If we are justified in applying the results of carefully controlled experimental work on monkeys and chimpanzees to man, we may say, in summary, that the premotor area is an important part of the extrapyramidal system for the control of postural reactions, and that destruction of this area or its projection system leads to spasticity as contrasted to the flaccidity which accompanies destructive lesions of the motor cortex. There are also certain reflex changes which appear to be characteristic of premotor deficiency, notably "forced grasping" and the "fanning" which occurs in the sign of Babinski.

4. The Motor Speech Area.—The function of speech, in its broader sense, is a most complex one and probably represents the highest activities of the human brain. The older notion that the speech centers were a series of compact compartments or centers located on the left side of the cerebrum in right-handed persons has been modified radically, like much of the other earlier work on cerebral localization. All recent work indicates that there is a widespread area on the left side of the brain concerned with the function of speech. This area includes the

lower part of the frontal and portions of the temporal and the parietal lobes (Fig. 22). The speech area has two great *incoming* paths—an *auditory* which enters the deep region of the temporal lobe, and a *visual* which enters near the angular gyrus. There is a great *outgoing* path to the motor cortex, and these fibers probably communicate with the *motor* speech center in the posterior third of the second and third frontal convolutions (Broca's area).

The handedness of the individual is a reliable index to the location of the functioning centers for speech. In the right-handed, the speech centers are on the left side of the brain, while in the left-handed, the reverse is true. No adequate explanation of this phenomenon has been made.

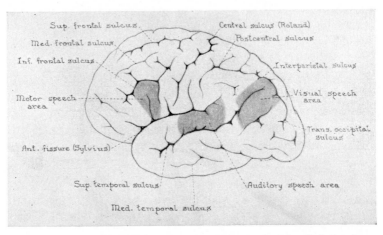

Fig. 22. Drawing of the lateral view of the left cerebral hemisphere, showing the important sulci and the cortical areas concerned with speech.

A lesion involving the speech area produces certain defects in verbation known as *aphasia*. Many varieties of aphasia have been described, but from the standpoint of cerebral localization only two need be considered—motor and sensory aphasia. Lesions situated anteriorly affect more markedly the execution of speech (motor), while those situated posteriorly disturb the reception of speech (sensory). The reader is referred to the section on the temporal lobe for a discussion of sensory aphasia.

The motor speech center (Broca's area) is located in the posterior third of the second and third frontal convolutions. Destruction of this area causes loss of ability to carry out the coördinated movements of the tongue, lips, pharynx, and larynx required in speaking. This area is not the direct cortical motor center for the muscles of speech; hence, in motor aphasia, there is no paralysis of these muscles.

Motor aphasia is clinically a true condition, although it is seldom seen without some involvement of the sensory speech mechanism. In its pure form, there is a loss of articulate speech without mental confusion or deterioration. If the motor speech area is destroyed, the patient is at first dumb. After a time, some degree of recovery ensues. Simple short words such as "yes," "no," "go," "eat," "cold," and "hot" are learned first. Then, he may learn to count or say the alphabet. He soon learns to construct short sentences. After many months of diligent work, he may acquire sufficient vocabulary to express his thoughts after a fashion. Difficult words are spoken badly if at all. He is apt to skip small words such as "in," "and," "an," etc., in making sentences. There is marked alteration of intonation and articulation. The tone of voice is monotonous and colorless. He often resorts to grimaces and gestures to express his thoughts. In spite of his difficulty of self expression, he has perfect comprehension of all auditory impulses. He may listen to the most involved conversation with perfect understanding.

CLINICAL. **Prefrontal Area.**—As already indicated in the physiological discussion of the frontal lobes, the left prefrontal lobe is the "master lobe" in right-handed individuals, the reverse being true in the left-handed. Consequently, it is most important to know whether a given patient is right- or left-handed. Handedness determines not only the dominant frontal lobe as far as higher psychic characteristics are concerned, but it also indicates the location of the speech areas.

The frontal lobes had been considered to be the "silent areas" of the brain until 1848 when study of the famous "crowbar case" shed light upon their activity. The patient was a Mr. P. P. Gage, a laborer, who was injured in an explosion, having had a crowbar driven through the left orbit into and through the left frontal lobe. He survived the injury for many years, and his chief occupation was placing himself and the crowbar on exhibition in many of the large medical centers. As the accident produced extensive destruction, he furnished an unusual opportunity for study of the effect of disease upon the dominant frontal lobe. The clinical changes observed were as follows:

1. Whereas, he had formerly been a man of even temperament and steady habits, he became subject to sudden unprovoked outbursts of rage; his moods were vacillating; he wandered aimlessly and had grandiose adventures.

2. His moral attitude showed a great change. Whereas formerly, he had been truthful, honest, and non-profane, he now became dishonest in his transactions, untruthful and excessively profane.

3. His judgment and reasoning ability became unreliable; consequently, he was always in difficulties wherever his wanderings led him.

He died 12 years after the injury in a severe convulsion.

Destructive lesions of the frontal lobes are characterized by varying degrees of memory loss and orientation, euphoria, and a change of habits. The memory loss is usually noticed first by the family or business associates of the patient. He becomes unreliable, often apathetic and indifferent. If disorientation occurs, he may be judged insane and committed to an institution for mental diseases. He is often unconcerned about his physical condition and, not infrequently, exhibits an exaggerated sense of well-being. He may develop an undue levity, persist in senseless joking and act in an undignified manner, out of keeping with his character as understood by his associates. He may be emotionally unstable and be subject to outbursts of crying. He may become slovenly in appearance, and, not infrequently, there are involuntary urination and defecation.

All of these manifestations are more prominent when the disease involves the dominant frontal lobe. In fact, it is not uncommon to observe destructive lesions of the right frontal lobe (in the right-handed) with no demonstrable mental changes.

True Motor Area.—Two types of symptom complexes develop as the result of disease involving the cortical motor area: (1) the syndrome of irritation; (2) the syndrome of destruction.

Irritative lesions cause paroxysmal attacks of local or diffuse spasms in the muscles corresponding to the affected areas. Thus, the face, upper extremity, trunk, or lower extremity may be involved independently of any other portion of the body. Usually, the spasm begins in one part, for instance, the muscles of the leg, and spreads in regular succession to the next adjacent part, until the entire half or even the whole body is involved in the convulsive seizure. This type of attack is known as a jacksonian convulsion and always indicates an organic lesion in the part of the motor cortex corresponding to the member which becomes involved first in the spasm. Loss of consciousness does not occur with a true jacksonian fit. A certain degree of paralysis, the duration of which may be only a few hours, usually follows this type of convulsion.

Destructive lesions produce loss of volitional control in the involved parts, the degree of which depends upon the extent of the destructive process and the time elapsing from the onset of symptoms. In acute lesions the paralysis is at first profound. With the lapse of time, there is gradual improvement in voluntary movement until perhaps 50 per cent is regained. The improvement is probably due to the opposite motor cortex and the extrapyramidal motor tracts taking over the functions of the destroyed areas. The paralysis is at first flaccid, i.e., the muscles are atonic and "flabby"; the tendon reflexes are absent, and the superficial reflexes are abolished. After a time, the muscles regain their tone and gradually become hypertonic with increased resistance to passive movement. The tendon reflexes then become hyperactive. In other words, a true state of spasticity ensues. Contractures in the paralyzed extremities are common.

If the onset of paralysis is more gradual, the flaccid stage is not observed; the paralysis is spastic from the beginning.

The first warning of impending paralysis is a feeling of awkwardness or weakness in the involved member. To demonstrate slight degrees of muscular weakness, the examiner should test each group of muscles separately by having the patient move them against resistance. Thus flexion and extension of the forearm are made against resistance provided by the examiner, the uninvolved arm of the patient being used for comparison. Spastic paralysis, involving the lower extremity, may sometimes be demonstrated by observing the tip of the shoe sole. A slight degree of toe-drop is of early occurrence; hence, the patient will drag his toe while walking, thus wearing off the tip of the sole on the involved side. For a more detailed discussion of the types of motor paralysis, the reader is referred to the section on the spinal cord.

Premotor Area.—When the region of the cortex which controls skilled acts (premotor area) becomes involved from disease or injury, the patient is no longer able to perform acts which he had acquired through repetition or application. For instance, if he attempts to write, the result will be imperfect or impossible, not because of muscle paralysis, for he may be able to produce a normal contraction in the individual muscle or groups of muscles required to execute the act. He apparently has lost the motion formula and is no longer able to transmit to the muscular tissue the pattern of motor impulses which controls the muscular contractions. This defect is known as motor apraxia.

Another interesting phenomenon associated with destructive lesions of the premotor area is "forced grasping." If the patient is asked to squeeze the examiner's fingers with both hands simultaneously and is suddenly commanded to "let go," the normal hand will obey the command promptly, but the hand contralateral to the lesion will continue to grasp the fingers. If the examiner makes an effort to release himself, the grip becomes firmer and firmer, and it may be several minutes before the patient is able to relax it.

This phenomenon probably represents a true reflex (palmar reflex) in which the inhibitory center has been removed by destruction of the premotor area in the contralateral frontal lobe. It may occur without evidence of pyramidal involvement; in fact, gross pyramidal involvement tends to abolish this reflex in man.

Motor Speech Center.—In testing for motor speech defects the examiner must distinguish clearly between an articular speech disturbance (dysarthria) and a non-articular speech defect (aphasia). The former is due to a defect in control of the *muscles* of speech—a form of asynergy. All words can be spoken, but the intonation and spacing of words are defective (see chapter on the cerebellum). In true motor aphasia, the patient will find it difficult or impossible to utter the right words in illustrating his thoughts.

In examining the aphasic patient, one first should establish definitely whether he is naturally right- or left-handed. Most children are taught to write with the right hand regardless of their natural handedness. The best index to handedness is obtained by inquiring with which hand he throws a ball, uses his fork in eating, etc., or, if a woman, with which hand she threads a needle, or combs her hair.

The following observations should then be made with regard to defects in motor speech:

1. Can the patient utter intelligible words spontaneously?

2. Is his vocabulary restricted to simple short words or sentences?

3. Can he pronounce all words or only a few?

4. Does he name objects correctly? Does he misplace words or syllables and, most important, does he recognize his errors and try to correct them?

If motor speech is involved primarily, defects as illustrated by the preceding questions will be found; at the same time, the patient will retain correct perception of auditory and visual sensations. In other words, he can respond to such commands as "smile," "whistle," "shut your eyes," etc.; also, he can understand such commands when written.

B. The Parietal Lobe

Anatomy and Physiology.—This region of the brain comprises a large part of the hemisphere. It is bounded in front by the Rolandic fissure, below by the Sylvian fissure and behind by an imaginary line, connecting the preoccipital notch with the external portion of the parieto-occipital fissure. Upon its lateral surface, the parietal lobe is divided by the interparietal and postcentral sulci into three convolutions: the postcentral, superior parietal and the inferior parietal gyri (Figs. 19, 22).

The functions of the whole parietal lobe have to do with receiving, arranging and elaborating sensory impulses which reach the brain through the various sensory systems of the body. Knowledge of the exact functions of the parietal lobe cortex is limited to the area comprising the postcentral convolution.

The postcentral convolution (sensory cortex) lies just posterior to the motor cortex, the two being separated by the Rolandic fissure. This area may be regarded as the region of the brain which serves as the primary receiving station of sensory impulses which enter into consciousness, a general assembling area of body sensations. Unlike the motor cortex, the sensory centers are not sharply limited. The general pattern conforms, however, to that which prevails in the motor area, the foot center being at the top and the face center at the bottom of the convolution. Because the corresponding sensory areas are more diffuse, more extensive destruction of the cortex is required to produce hypesthesia of the arm than paralysis of the arm.

Just posterior to the sensory cortex lies the intermediate postcentral area (psychosensory). This zone of cortex holds an intimate relation to the postcentral area and serves in the capacity of elaborating the sensory impulses received by the primary sensory area, so that they attain their full usefulness. This process may be compared to cataloging, in that the cerebral activities are selected and filed in proper relation to other sensory impulses having the same general character.

The functions of the remainder of the parietal lobe, i.e., the extensive area between the temporal, postcentral, and occipital areas, are for the most part obscure. Apparently, in the superior parietal convolution is a center for the association of memories of form, or more properly for the perception of the form of objects. When this region is destroyed, astereognosis (loss of perception of form) results. On the inferior parietal convolution, on the left side in right-handed individuals, there is an area concerned with memory of written words (reading center). In this same region, there is perhaps a center for memories concerning the use of things (praxic center).

CLINICAL.—Acute destructive lesions of the postcentral convolution produce profound sensory loss in the contralateral half of the body. All forms of sensation may be lost (anesthesia) if the destruction is complete. Recovery of certain forms of sensation is rapid and after a few weeks it may be difficult to demonstrate any loss of pain, heat and cold and touch sensibility. However, stereognostic sense, two-point discrimination, and position sense remain badly impaired permanently. The patient may complain severely of a numb sensation involving an arm; he may drop objects which he attempts to pick up, or he may burn himself before feeling the sensation of heat. This type of sensory abnormality is characteristic of cortical lesions in contradistinction to loss of sensation resulting from involvement of the sensory tracts in the peripheral nerves, spinal cord or brain-stem. (For methods of sensory examination see section on spinal cord.)

Irritative lesions of the sensory cortex produce in the contralateral half of the body a sensation not far removed from pain, most frequently described as "pins and needles." Such sensory disturbances commonly comprise the "aura" preceding an attack of jacksonian epilepsy and are unusual except with a convulsive discharge. The site at which the sensory aura begins indicates the cortical location of the lesion.

Lesions in the region of the superior parietal convolution produce, in addition to superficial sensory disturbances, a condition known as *astereognosis*. The patient is no longer able to differentiate or appreciate the form, size or consistency of objects placed in his hand. In testing for astereognosis, the patient, with his eyes closed, is asked to identify such objects as a key, knife or coin placed in his hand by the examiner. The inability to identify them by palpation indicates a loss of stereognostic sense, the defect being called *astereognosis*.

C. The Occipital Lobe

ANATOMY.—The occipital lobe is situated at the posterior pole of each hemisphere. Only a small portion of the lateral surface of the hemisphere is formed by this lobe (Fig. 19). On the mesial surface, the lobe forms a long triangular field between the parietal lobe anteriorly and the temporal lobe inferiorly (Fig. 23). Mesially, it is divided into two parts by the calcarine fissure: the cuneus, and the lingual gyrus. This fissure begins vertical to the splenium of the corpus callosum and extends toward the occipital pole. The visual centers are located in the cortex, forming the wall of the calcarine fissure, and in the adjacent portions of the cuneus, and lingual gyrus.

The occipital lobe is more nearly a structural and functional entity than any of the other lobes. All of its functions are concerned directly or indirectly with visual processes.

The special sense of sight has two centers: the primary and the secondary. The primary center is in the lateral geniculate body. The secondary center is situated in the occipital lobe particularly upon the mesial surface in and about the calcarine fissure. Each occipital lobe is the center for visual impulses from the corresponding half of the retina of each eye (Fig. 2).

For a more complete description of the visual pathways, the reader is referred to the section on the optic nerve, page 17.

CLINICAL.—Irritative lesions of the calcarine area produce visual hallucinations, usually characterized as "flashing of light" or "sheet lightning" (see page 19).

The impairment or destruction of the entire calcarine area of one side produces blindness in the opposite visual field (homonymous hemianopsia). If only a part of one calcarine area is destroyed, an homonymous field defect, corresponding to the involved visual fibers, results. The superior quadrants of the retina are represented in the upper portion of the calcarine fissure. The lower quadrants have their centers in the lower calcarine area. Thus, if only the upper calcarine area is involved, an inferior quadrant homonymous field defect occurs (Fig. 6).

For methods of examination and the interpretation of visual defects, see page 20.

D. THE TEMPORAL LOBE

ANATOMY.—On its external surface, the temporal lobe is divided into three well-defined convolutions: the superior, middle and inferior temporal gyri (Fig. 22). It is separated from the frontal and parietal lobes by the Sylvian fissure. The ventral surface of the lobe lies on the floor of the middle fossa of the skull. A fourth temporal gyrus, which is situated between the inferior temporal sulcus and the collateral fissure, appears on the ventral surface. This gyrus is commonly called the temporosphenoidal convolution.

The dorsal surface of the temporal lobe is concealed from view in the depths of the Sylvian fissure. In order to bring this surface of the lobe into view, it is necessary to excise the portions of the frontal and parietal lobes which conceal it. When these portions of the hemisphere are removed, two or three prominent convolutions are found to mark the dorsal surface of the lobe. These are the transverse gyri of Heschl and represent the cortical center of hearing.

On the mesial surface of the temporal lobe are seen the prominent uncinate and hippocampal gyri. The cortical centers for the sense of smell and perhaps taste are located in these gyri (Fig. 23).

CLINICAL.—The right temporal lobe in the right-handed is a relatively "silent" area of the brain. Aside from cortical centers of hearing and smell, no definite localization of function is known to exist in this region. The left temporal lobe, in addition to harboring cortical centers for hearing and smell, contains the important association tracts and centers concerned with speech.

Since the ear is bilaterally represented in the cerebral cortex, the destruction of one auditory center does not produce unilateral deafness. Unilateral lesions will, however, produce dullness in acuity of hearing equally in both ears. (See section on the auditory nerve.)

Irritative lesions in the region of the uncinate and hippocampal gyri cause hallucinations of smell and taste, the so-called *"uncinate fit."* This symptom is of great importance in the diagnosis of expanding lesions of the temporal lobe (see section on the olfactory nerve).

"Dreamy state" is a queer phenomenon which occurs frequently in temporal lobe tumors or abscesses. During one of

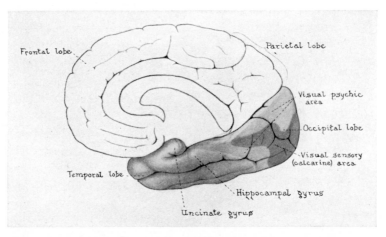

FIG. 23. Cerebral cortex—mesial surface. Shaded areas show the important landmarks of the occipital and temporal lobes.

these periods, the patient feels as though his surroundings are unreal or far away, yet at the same time curiously familiar. He is aroused from this attitude with difficulty. Sometimes this dreamy state may pass into one of extreme drowsiness which may last for several days without interruption. No anatomical data are available to account for this phenomenon.

The optic radiations pass through the substance of the temporal lobe, the fibers being drawn out in a loop as they sweep around the temporal horn of the lateral ventricle. Consequently, lesions of the temporal lobe may block the transmission of impulses from the corresponding half of each retina and, thus, an homonymous hemianopsia, or at least an homonymous visual field defect will result (Fig. 6). Study of the visual fields is of paramount importance in the recognition of temporal lobe tumors and abscesses.

Sensory Aphasia.—The function of speech seems to be composed of at least two component parts—sensory and motor. The sensory portion is concerned with incoming impulses to the speech area by way of the auditory, visual, and kinesthetic pathways. The motor portion represents the outgoing pathways from the speech area to the motor cortex. The cortical areas concerned with sensory speech are closely related to the cortical centers for hearing, sight and kinesthetic sense. However, these cortical representations for speech are unilateral; in the right-handed, they are on the left side of the brain, the reverse being true in the left-handed.

Lesions of the left temporal lobe in the right-handed produce disorders of speech in which auditory stimuli lack comprehension. The patient hears the spoken word but no longer understands its meaning. He uses words incorrectly, plurals instead of singulars, or masculine instead of feminine pronouns, probably because the sound perception of his own speech is defective. He has difficulty in naming objects correctly and is unaware of his errors. He seems to have lost the memory for the sound of words. In contrast to the patient with motor aphasia, he may speak fluently, but unless he confines his speech to conventional phrasing, he commits grave errors in the use of words.

Lesions in the region of the angular gyrus (near the junction of the parietal, temporal and occipital lobes) produce another characteristic type of aphasia commonly known as *word blindness*. The patient is unable to recognize the meaning of written or printed words. He is unable to write because he cannot "see" or comprehend what he is writing. He is unable to read, not because of blindness, but because he lacks visual comprehension. His speech otherwise may not be affected. Since the optic radiations are close by, word blindness is usually associated with right homonymous hemianopsia (see page 18).

Pure types of motor or sensory aphasia are distinctly rare. Lesions of the speech areas are usually sufficiently large to depress the speech faculty as a whole. However, if the expressive (motor) side of speech is more involved, the lesion lies anteriorly in the frontotemporal region, while if the appreciative (sensory) side of speech shows the greater impairment, the lesion lies posteriorly in the temporoparietal lobe.

E. The Corpus Striatum

Situated deeply in the substance of each cerebral hemisphere is a group of nuclei collectively known as the basal ganglia. Two of these masses of gray matter, the caudate and lenticular nuclei, constitute the *corpus striatum*.

The importance of this structure to clinical neurology is due to the fact that lesions of it produce a group of symptoms unlike those arising from any other part of the brain.

Anatomy.—The corpus striatum is situated near the base of each cerebral hemisphere. It consists of a large oval mass of gray matter embedded in the white substance of the hemisphere, a portion of which (caudate nucleus) is visible in the frontal horn of the lateral ventricle (Fig. 24).

The caudate nucleus is the more mesial portion of the corpus striatum. It is an elongated mass composed of a large head, a long slender body and a slender tail. The whole structure is

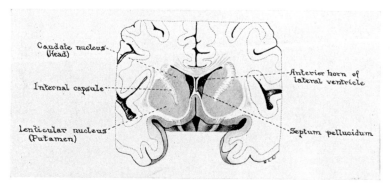

Fig. 24. Drawing of a cross section of the brain at the level of the anterior end of the corpus striatum.

bent upon itself like a horseshoe. At its anterior-most part, the caudate nucleus is fused with the lenticular nucleus. It is separated from this structure posterior to the fused area by the internal capsule.

The lenticular nucleus, the larger of the two masses, is subdivided into an external part, the *putamen* and an internal part, the *globus pallidus*. The globus is composed of many groups of large multipolar and pyramidal shaped cells, resembling somewhat the anterior horn cells. The caudate nucleus and putamen are composed chiefly of small oval cells like those found in the sensory centers.

The various connections of the corpus striatum are still imperfectly understood. The caudate nucleus is closely connected by afferent fibers with the thalamus. Communicating fibers join together the various parts of the corpus striatum. The majority of these run from the caudate nucleus to the putamen and from there to the globus pallidus. All the efferent fibers of the corpus striatum arise in the globus pallidus and are distributed through the ansa lenticularis to the red nucleus, substantia nigra, hypothalamic nucleus and the thalamus (Fig. 25).

The corpus striatum has few, if any, connections with the cerebral cortex. All of its afferent impulses are received from the thalamus, and all of its efferent fibers arise in the globus

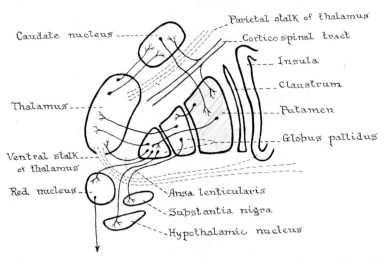

FIG. 25. Diagram illustrating the probable connections of the caudate and lenticular nuclei. (After Ranson)

pallidus. Thus, the globus pallidus may be regarded as a part of the motor mechanism of the brain, and the caudate nucleus and putamen, through their connections with the thalamus, exert some controlling influence upon this motor mechanism. The centers in the mid and hind-brain, to which the fibers from the globus pallidus connect, give rise to a series of motor tracts called the *extrapyramidal* tracts. These motor tracts have their cells of origin at a subcortical level. They play an important part in the regulation and maintenance of bodily posture.

CLINICAL.—Most of the experimental work upon the functions of the corpus striatum in lower animals is not applicable to man. As the development of the cerebral cortex increases in the ascent of the animal scale, the function of the corpus striatum steadily decreases. In proportion to the bulk of the brain, the corpus striatum is considerably smaller in man than in other animals, and its functions have, to a corresponding degree, been taken over by the higher cortical centers. In birds, for instance, the pyramidal tracts are absent, and the corpus striatum may be wholly responsible for voluntary movement.

In man, it is extremely doubtful whether or not it controls any sort of voluntary movement.

The effect of disease upon the corpus striatum provides us with our only knowledge of its function in man. The principal disorders observed are:

1. Muscular rigidity.
2. Tremor—involuntary movements.
3. Slowing of voluntary movements.
4. Change in emotional expression.

1. Muscular Rigidity.—Rigidity is constantly present and is almost universal in its distribution. The muscles are firm, tense and show excessive resistance to passive motion. The limbs usually occupy a position of flexion due to the fact that the flexor groups are stronger than the extensors. Contractures sooner or later develop. A characteristic attitude often results from the contractures of the flexor groups. The head is bent on the chest; the back is slightly flexed; the arms are adducted and flexed, and the knees bent. The rigidity is often so marked that the patient can be moved about *en bloc* like a statue.

2. Tremor and Involuntary Movements.—Tremor is frequently the initial symptom of disease of the corpus striatum. It occurs when the limbs are at rest (non-intentional tremor) and is exaggerated by voluntary movement (intentional tremor). The tremor varies from a very fine to a coarse movement. It is, as a rule, of a slow rate, averaging about six contractions per second. It is modified by varying conditions. During sleep, it disappears, and during emotional excitement, it is increased. The tremor usually appears first in the flexors and extensors of the fingers, next in the supinators and pronators of the arm. Occasionally, however, the tremor is first observed in the neck muscles or in the tongue. Later the tremor may spread gradually to all the voluntary musculature.

It should not be implied that tremors are pathognomonic of disease of the corpus striatum. They may occur in connection with other diseases, notably cerebellar dysfunction and hyperthyroidism. However, the rhythmic tremors that accompany striatal disease are, as a rule, more pronounced than those seen in any other pathological state.

3. Slowing of Voluntary Movements.—Voluntary movements are slow, irregular and limited in extent in striatal disease. All the smaller muscles, especially those of the hand, are affected. Clumsiness and inability to perform fine movements are two of the early symptoms. The muscles of articulation and phonation are both impaired. Weakness of the lips, soft palate and tongue results in a "slurring" type of speech. Immobility of the larynx causes extreme monotony of the voice. There is relative weakness of the muscles, and fatigue sets in more rapidly than normally.

The larger groups of muscles are less affected in this regard than are the smaller muscles. However, all the muscles, regardless of their size, show a lessened range, lessened flexibility and a slowness of reaction.

When the patient is at rest, he sits still and does not indulge in spontaneous movements, such as crossing the legs, as does a normal person. He seems to lack the desire to move.

The gait is slow and "shuffling." The patient does not swing his arms when walking.

4. Changes in Emotional Expression.—In lesions of the corpus striatum, the face is "mask-like" in appearance. All emotional movements are carried out slowly and ineffectively. He can, however, laugh and cry, but even these emotional states do not appear to be genuine because of his immobile facial expression.

All of the evidence of functional activity of the corpus striatum in man has been derived from clinical and pathological data. That all the phenomena listed above are due solely to a sharply localized lesion of the caudate and lenticular nuclei is still a controversial subject. However, we may safely say that the structure is one of the centers which controls tone in skeletal muscles, and that its injury results in an excess of muscle tone characterized by rigidity, tremor and certain disorders of voluntary motion.

There are three well established clinical syndromes associated with disease of the corpus striatum:

1. Paralysis agitans (Parkinson's disease).
2. Encephalitis lethargica (postencephalitic parkinsonism).
3. Progressive lenticular degeneration (Wilson's disease).

The first two syndromes are very similar in their clinical manifestations, the most important distinguishing feature being that paralysis agitans is a disease of old age, while encephalitic parkinsonism is seen usually in young adults.

Epidemic encephalitis with its sequelae has rendered the parkinsonian syndrome all too common. Whether the symptoms result from epidemic encephalitis or from vascular disease of the brain (paralysis agitans), the chief lesion encountered at autopsy is degeneration and destruction of the substance and the connecting pathways of the corpus striatum.

A typical advanced Parkinson's syndrome consists of:

1. A characteristic attitude best described as one of general flexion.
2. A "mask-like" face, staring and expressionless.
3. Muscular hypertonia and rigidity.
4. Slowing of voluntary movements with weakness and increased fatigability.
5. Disorder or paralysis of conjugate vertical and horizontal ocular movements.
6. Impairment of articulation and phonation.
7. A slow, "shuffling" gait, often associated with propulsion and retropulsion.
8. Tremors, either intentional, non-intentional, or both are invariably present.
9. Mental changes in the terminal stages.

There are certain clinical differences between paralysis agitans and encephalitic parkinsonism. Tremor, for instance, is the most prominent symptom in the former, rigidity in the latter. Movements of the jaw, face and tongue are early symptoms of the syndrome following encephalitis, while these parts are involved only in the terminal stages of paralysis agitans. Moreover, a history of an acute attack of encephalitis is obtainable in the vast majority of the cases of encephalitic parkinsonism.

Oculogyric crises are very common in postencephalitic parkinsonism but are seldom seen in paralysis agitans. Such attacks consist of violent movement of the eyes upward or to one side associated with marked emotional distress, turning of the head backward, forward, or to the side, and often with propulsion or retropulsion if the patient is standing at the onset of the attack. In many instances the attack ends in sleep. Emotional excitement usually precipitates the attack and any existing tremors are always intensified.

Wilson's disease (progressive lenticular degeneration) occurs in childhood and is characterized by:

1. Muscular hypertonicity and rigidity.
2. Tremor.
3. Dysarthria and dysphagia.
4. Muscular weakness and emaciation.
5. Hypertrophic cirrhosis of the liver.
6. The occurrence of the disease in adolescence.
7. A familial and hereditary tendency.
8. Absence of sensory loss or evidence of pyramidal tract involvement.
9. Absence of psychic changes.

Other less clear-cut syndromes of this region of the brain have been described, but the ones listed above suffice to indicate the salient features of striatal disease.

CHAPTER IV

THE CEREBELLUM

ANATOMY.—The cerebellum, pons and medulla oblongata are housed in the posterior cranial fossa, separated from the cerebral hemispheres and the midbrain by a partition of dura called the tentorium cerebelli. Thus, the contents of the posterior fossa are connected with the contents of the anterior and middle cranial fossae only by a small opening in the tentorium (incisura) at a point where the pons joins with the midbrain.

The cerebellum may be divided into three parts: the median portion called the vermis, and two larger lateral masses, the

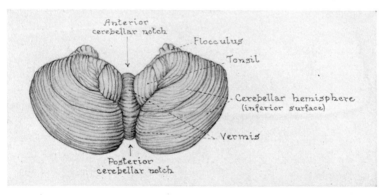

FIG. 26. Anterior view of the human cerebellum.
(After Sobotta-McMurrich)

cerebellar hemispheres, which are connected with each other by the vermis.

The cerebellum is composed of a thin superficial layer of gray matter, spread over an irregular white center that contains several separate nuclear masses. The cortex is folded to form many slender convolutions, separated by parallel sulci (Fig. 26). The white matter is formed in large part by fibers which enter and leave the cerebellum through its three peduncles.

The largest of the three peduncles is the middle one (brachium pontis). It is composd of fibers which after synapse in the pontine nuclei carry impulses from the cerebral cortex of the opposite side. The superior cerebellar peduncle (brachium conjunctivum) consists of fibers connecting the cerebellum with the red nucleus and thalamus of the opposite side. The inferior cerebellar peduncle (restiform body) consists of ascending fibers from the spinal cord and medulla oblongata. Thus, the cerebellum is intimately connected with the motor pathways which supply the whole skeletal muscular system and the great sensory pathways, especially those whose end-organs are in muscles, tendons and joints. It is to be remembered that each cerebellar hemisphere supplies the homolateral extremities as a result of two decussations—one afferent and one efferent —through the red nucleus.

PHYSIOLOGY.—The fundamental function of the cerebellum is synergy, i.e., the faculty with which complex movements are performed smoothly and synchronously. Thus, the muscular correlation required to carry out movements of different parts of the same limb, or of the limbs, head and trunk together, constitutes one example of synergy or synergic movement.

From the standpoint of functional development, the cerebellum may properly be regarded as a highly specialized vestibular nucleus. Certainly, the functions of the vestibular apparatus and the cerebellum are so intimately related, that it is often difficult to distinguish between symptoms which are purely vestibular and those that are purely cerebellar. In view of the extensive anatomical connections between the labyrinths and the cerebellum, we may assume that they work together for the production of synergic muscular movements, maintenance of equilibrium and the coördination of reflex tonic muscular activities.

There have been many efforts made to demonstrate localization of function in the different parts of the cerebellum. Aside from the generally accepted fact that the left hemisphere controls the synergic actions of the muscles on the left half of the body, and the right hemisphere those on the right side, the attempts at finer localization have not been convincing.

The first important experimental work upon the function of the cerebellum was by Flourens in 1824. His observations were made on pigeons after removing the organ entirely or in part. The most striking result from complete removal was a total inability to stand or move, even though there seemed to be no muscular paralysis. The animals seemed to lack completely the power to coördinate properly the contractions of the various muscles involved in maintaining equilibrium. When the experimental lesion was less extensive, the animals exhibited a staggering, drunken gait, and a decided uncertainty in all their movements. He was led by the striking results of his operations to suggest the view that the cerebellum is an organ for the coördination of movements and locomotion.

Many objections have been raised to this view, most important of which arise from the work of Luciani. He performed experiments upon dogs and monkeys. After completely removing the cerebellum, he found that the animal passed through three distinct stages: 1. that of functional exaltation; 2. that of maximum cerebellar deficiency; 3. that of compensation and partial recovery.

1. In this stage the animal is agitated and exhibits opisthotonos, head retraction and tonic extension and abduction of the forelimbs, with clonic movements of the hind-limbs. There is a staggering gait and frequently a horizontal nystagmus. He assumes that this stage is caused by the sudden removal of tonic inhibitory impulses which normally proceed from the cerebellum. No symptoms comparable to these have been observed in man.

2. The second stage consists of hypotonia, astasia and asthenia. Hypotonia implies a general reduction of postural tonus; astasia, a loss of steadiness in muscular movements which produces a staggering gait and tremors; asthenia, an abnormal tendency to fatigue with a loss of force in the muscular contractions.

3. The third stage is one in which the animal reacquires the

ability to stand and walk. The gait is at first extremely un-
steady, but he soon learns to walk with a wide base. The picture
is that of cerebellar ataxia. He explains the improvement on
the assumption that the cerebrum gradually takes over cerebellar functions.

According to Luciani then, the functions of the cerebellum
are concerned with the maintenance of tone in the body musculature, to maintain the steadiness of that tone and to increase
the energy of muscular movements.

The symptoms of cerebellar lesions in man are, on the whole,
very consistent with those produced experimentally in animals,
especially those in monkeys and dogs. A patient in whom the
cerebellum has been largely destroyed by a neoplasm exhibits
marked lack of coördination or synergetic control. He staggers
when he walks. Muscular tremors develop during voluntary
motion. He shows a lack of skill and speed in performing movements which require the associated activity of several muscles,
for example, the placing of the finger tip to the nose or the
rapid alternation in contraction of antagonistic muscles, like
pronation and supination. His muscular contractions are weak,
and he fatigues easily. When he speaks, the voice is drawling
and expressionless, and the words are slurred or jerked out
explosively. After a lesion of the sort just described has been
removed, even though there has been very extensive destruction
of cerebellar tissue, the symptoms gradually improve, and in
the course of time may be sufficiently insignificant to interfere
but little with the activities of the individual.

CLINICAL.—The signs and symptoms of cerebellar disease
are:

1. Disorders of station and gait.
2. Hypotonia.
3. Ataxia or asynergy.
4. Nystagmus.
5. Dysarthria.

When cerebellar disease causes interference with the circulation of cerebrospinal fluid, the following signs and symptoms are likely to develop in addition to those enumerated above:

1. Headache.
2. Vomiting.
3. Double vision.
4. Papilloedema.

Disorders of *station* and *gait* are perhaps the most characteristic features of cerebellar disease. If the lesion be an extensive one, the patient is unable to stand without support, there being a tendency to fall toward the affected side as though drawn by a magnet. If the lesion be in the midline (vermis), there is a tendency for the patient to fall backward or forward. In less severe cases, when the patient is able to stand unsupported, the slightest push toward the affected side will send him sprawling. The head is frequently inclined toward the affected side and held in a fixed position while standing. Any voluntary movement of the head tends to exaggerate the unstable station.

In testing for an abnormal station, the patient should stand erect with feet together. If the incoördination is severe, he will fall toward the affected side; if less severe, he will sway and attempt to throw his weight on the sound leg. When there is exaggeration of swaying with the eyes closed, a positive Romberg sign is said to be present. This sign is characteristic of diseases which involve the dorsal column of the spinal cord, notably, tabes and combined sclerosis. However, swaying in purely cerebellar disease is usually intensified by closing the eyes.

Some degree of staggering gait is always present in cerebellar disease. However, staggering gait occurs in lesions of other localities, particularly those involving the labyrinth and the posterior columns of the spinal cord. It is not uncommon for patients with cerebellar tumor to give a history of having been arrested for intoxication because of the reeling gait which they exhibit while walking. When the lesion is an extensive one, the patient tries to preserve his equilibrium by standing on a wide base with his legs well abducted. Even then, he is apt to sway and totter. As stated previously, when the lesion is chiefly unilateral, the patient tends to reel or stagger toward the affected side. When testing for a staggering gait, the patient is asked to walk in a straight line. If the incoördination is of slight degree, walking with one foot placed immediately in front of the other (tandem) will often demonstrate an unstable gait which otherwise would escape notice.

By *hypotonia*, is meant a lack of tone in the muscles, especially those of the limbs. Some degree of this phenomenon is present in nearly every case of cerebellar disease. Hypotonia may be demonstrated in many ways. Perhaps the simplest test consists of shaking an affected limb and observing that the excursions are limited only by the ligaments and joints, whereas the excursions of a normal limb are checked to a certain degree by muscle tone. Another test for hypotonia is the rebound phenomenon of Gordon-Holmes. The patient is asked to pull his forearm upward against the resistance offered by the examiner. Normally, when the resistance is suddenly removed, the excursion of the forearm is soon arrested by contraction of the antagonistic group of muscles. In cerebellar disease, when the resistance is suddenly removed, the forearm flies upward toward the face without any effort on the part of the antagonistic group of muscles to check the force of the upward movement. With lesions of one-half of the cerebellum, the hypotonia is confined to the same side of the body.

Some degree of *cerebellar ataxia* or *asynergy* is universally present in diseases affecting this part of the brain. By ataxia, we mean the inability to control the coördinate movements of muscles. By asynergy, we mean the lack of coördination between parts normally acting in harmony.

Every simple voluntary movement is a very complex action involving several groups of muscles. First of all, there is contraction or shortening of the muscle or group of muscles immediately concerned in the movement. Simultaneously, the antagonistic group either relaxes to facilitate the movement or contracts to render the movement steady or to prevent its exaggeration. In addition, other groups of muscles fix the joints in relation to the moving parts. All of these muscle groups require a background of postural tonus for proper execution of the voluntary movement; otherwise, it will be poorly coördinated, tremulous and jerky. In cerebellar disorders, postural tonus of this sort is lacking; hence, voluntary movements become ataxic and asynergic.

There are many clinical tests for ataxia and asynergy. The ones given below are those in common usage and suffice to demonstrate any significant degree of these phenomena.

(a) **Finger-to-Nose Test.**—With the patient standing in the erect position, he is asked to touch the tip of the nose with the tip of the index finger, the outstretched upper extremity being placed in various positions by the examiner. He performs the test several times with either hand, first with the eyes open, and then with the eyes closed. The examiner observes the smoothness of the motion and its accuracy both with the eyes open and closed. In cerebellar disease, the movement of the arm is jerky and tremulous. Frequently, the tip of the finger will not reach the tip of the nose, or else it will overshoot the mark. Closing the eyes, as a rule, exaggerates the ataxia. If the lesion is confined to one cerebellar hemisphere, the ataxia is limited to the same side.

(b) **Finger-to-Finger Test.**—With the arms outstretched, the tips of the index fingers are brought together in front of the patient. Then, the extended arms are drawn backward as far as possible. The patient then attempts to touch the tips of the index fingers together with a slow unhurried motion of the arms forward. After two attempts of this sort with the eyes open, the test is repeated with the eyes closed. A normal person can accomplish this test accurately with the eyes either open or closed, but the patient with cerebellar disease will miss the mark whether the eyes are open or closed. If the lesion be a unilateral one, the ipsilateral arm will sag and undershoot the finger on the normal side.

(c) **Finger-to-Thumb Test.**—With the patient standing erect he is asked to extend the upper extremities and rapidly approximate the fingers to the thumbs in sequence. If ataxia is present on one or both sides, the movements will be performed awkwardly, and after correctly approximating two or three fingers to the thumb, he will become "mixed up" and the voluntary movements will cease.

(d) **Past-Pointing Test.**—With the patient and the examiner either seated or standing facing each other, the outstretched upper extremity of each is held in a horizontal position, so that their index fingers are in contact. Then, the patient is asked to elevate his arm to a vertical position, so that the finger is pointed directly upward. Then, he attempts to return the arm to the horizontal position in such a way that his index finger will again come in contact with that of the examiner's. This motion should be performed slowly and with deliberation. After two or three attempts with the eyes open, the test should be tried with the eyes closed. Each upper extremity is examined separately. A normal person performs this test without deviation of the finger to one side or the other. A patient with cerebellar or acute labyrinthian defects will invariably past-point in the test, and with the eyes closed, the error will usually be greater.

(e) **Heel-to-Knee Test.**—This test is used for demonstrating ataxia in the lower extremities. It is performed only in the recumbent position. The patient is asked to place the heel of one foot upon the knee of the other leg and push the heel along the shin to the foot in a straight line. First one leg then the other is tested with the eyes open and closed. If ataxia or asynergy is present, the heel will often overshoot or undershoot the knee, and when once the descent along the shin is started, the heel will "jump the track" or else be pushed downward with a series of jerks. This test is especially important in certain cerebellar lesions when coördination in the upper extremities is nearly normal.

(f) **Adiadokokinesis.**—The test for adiadokokinesis is usually performed by having the patient rapidly pronate and supinate the outstretched hands. However, any simple movement with the two corresponding limbs, performed rapidly, will demonstrate this defect when present. In unilateral cerebellar disease, the disorders of range and rate of movements on the affected side contrast vividly with the regular, coördinated movements of the sound limb. The rate on the affected side is much slower than normal; the movements are very irregular, there being an appreciable interval between pronation and supination, and if the effort continues, the movements may cease abruptly. When the test is performed with the affected limb only, adiadokokinesis is less apparent, because the patient is able to give his undivided attention to the one limb.

Nystagmus is nearly always present in cerebellar disease. However, one occasionally sees cases of cerebellar tumor where one hemisphere is practically destroyed by the growth, without any trace of nystagmus. The mechanism of nystagmus and the test for its presence have already been discussed (page 34). For sake of emphasis, it should be repeated that nystagmus consists of a quick phase in the direction of the voluntary movements of the eyes, followed by a slow phase in which the eyes return to the position of rest. Usually, the quick phase is more marked when the gaze is directed toward the side of the lesion. The essential component of nystagmus is the slow phase which implies a failure of the eyes to maintain a position into which they were voluntarily moved. This phenomenon in cerebellar disease may, therefore, be regarded as a deficiency of tonus in the muscles which maintain the position of the eyes, i.e., a true hypotonia.

Disorders of speech are commonly observed in cerebellar disease. Articulation and phonation are dependent upon coördinated contractions of various muscle groups; therefore, it is to be expected that in cerebellar disease, defects in speech would occur, since the fundamental disorder is asynergy. The tone of the voice may be monotonous and drawling. Syllables are separated from each other by unnatural intervals, or the words may be jerked out explosively. Often the words are slurred together so that the speech may be unintelligible. The muscles of articulation fatigue easily, and what at first may be considered normal speech, after a few minutes of conversation may become decidedly defective. Lesions involving the vermis are more commonly associated with speech disorders.

Space-occupying lesions of the cerebellum (tumors and abscesses) often produce, in addition to the true cerebellar symptomatology, symptoms of increased intracranial pressure from interference with the flow of cerebrospinal fluid. With tumors situated in the vermis, the first symptoms may be those of obstructive hydrocephalus. Referring again to the anatomical discussion at the beginning of this chapter, one recalls that the contents of the posterior fossa of the skull consist of the cerebellum, pons and medulla oblongata; that the posterior fossa is a closed cavity, with the exception of the incisura of the cerebellar tentorium above and the foramen magnum below. The only means of escape of the cerebrospinal fluid from the ventricular system in the brain is from the roof and lateral recesses of the fourth ventricle in the medulla oblongata. The vermis of the cerebellum lies immediately upon the fourth ventricle. With these facts in mind, it becomes obvious why expanding lesions of this region should so frequently block the escape of cerebrospinal fluid, thereby producing an obstructive internal hydrocephalus.

Headache is usually the first symptom of obstruction. It is severe from the onset and is generalized as a rule. As the pressure increases, *vomiting* usually occurs. The vomiting may be projectile and is often unassociated with nausea. *Double vision* frequently makes its appearance after the onset of the headache and vomiting. This is due to sixth nerve paralysis on one or both sides, resulting from damage by the highly increased intracranial pressure to the nerve in its course to the orbit. *Papilloedema* (choked disc) develops often within a few days after the onset of the obstructive hydrocephalus. As a rule, the papilloedema progresses rapidly, and damage to vision occurs quickly unless the obstruction is relieved. It is not uncommon to see patients completely blind within three or four weeks after the first symptoms of obstruction from cerebellar tumor.

CHAPTER V

THE SPINAL CORD

ANATOMY AND PHYSIOLOGY.—The spinal cord is a cylindrical mass of nervous tissue housed in the canal of the vertebral column. In the human embryo of 3 months, it occupies the entire length of the vertebral canal, and the spinal nerves pass lateralward to their exit through the intervertebral foramina. As growth occurs, the vertebral column increases in length more rapidly than the spinal cord, and as a result, the cord ends in the adult at the lower border of the first or upper border of the second lumbar vertebra. Consequently, the nerve roots run in a caudal direction from their points of origin to the same intervertebral foramina through which they made their exit before the cord shifted its position (Fig. 27). Since the cord ends at the level of the first and second lumbar vertebrae, the roots of the lumbar, sacral, and coccygeal nerves, in order to reach their proper foramina, descend vertically in the canal, forming a large bundle called the *cauda equina*. The cord ends above at its junction with the medulla oblongata at the level of the foramen magnum. The cord is covered by a continuation of the three membranes of the brain, the dura, the arachnoid and the pia. The membranes descend to the third sacral vertebra or lower. The cord is suspended in its dural sac by the dentate ligaments. One process of this ligament is found between each pair of spinal roots down to the first lumbar segment where the ligaments end (Fig. 27). The cord and its membranes are protected in the bony canal by a thick cushion of adipose tissue.

The size of the cord is not uniform throughout, the cervical and lumbar portions being larger than the thoracic portion. The cervical and lumbar enlargements result from increase in gray matter necessary for the innervation of the extremities. The time of the first appearance and the subsequent growth of these enlargements are directly related to the development of the limbs (Fig. 27).

For purposes of description, the spinal cord is divided into segments. Each segment embraces that portion which gives rise to a pair of spinal nerves. There are thirty-one pairs of

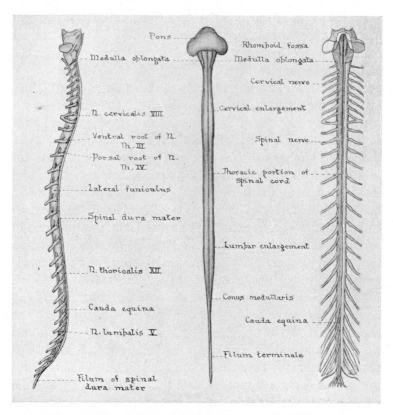

FIG. 27. Three views of the spinal cord and brain-stem.
(After Ranson-Spalteholz)

spinal nerves; eight are cervical, twelve thoracic, five lumbar, five sacral, and one coccygeal. From each segment throughout the length of the cord, arise bilaterally a posterior root (sensory) and an anterior root (motor) which in turn join to form the spinal nerve (Fig. 28).

A cross section of the spinal cord shows two kinds of tissue, white and gray. The white substance, which forms a thick mantle surrounding the gray matter, is composed of myelinated and unmyelinated fibers supported by a framework of neuroglia. Groups of these fibers associated functionally and anatomically constitute the fiber tracts. The centrally placed gray substance is made up of nerve cells including their dendrites, unmyelinated axons, a few myelinated fibers, and many blood vessels, all supported by a network of neuroglia (Fig. 28).

To obtain a proper understanding of the finer anatomy of the

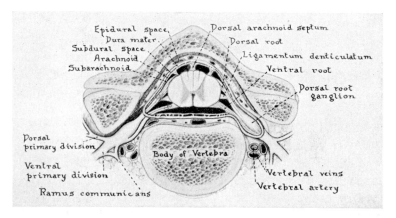

FIG. 28. Transverse section through the vertebral column, showing the relationship between the cord, nerve roots, meninges, vertebral vessels, and bony parts of the vertebra. (Tilney and Riley—Rauber)

spinal cord, one must think of it in terms of function as well as structure. The spinal cord as an organ has two great functions to perform. First, through a system of reflex centers, the activities of glands, blood vessels, visceral organs and, to a degree, the voluntary muscular system are controlled. Second, through its system of fiber tracts, a mechanism is provided for the conduction of impulses to and from the brain. The first of these spinal cord functions—the spinal reflex mechanism—will be dealt with in the next chapter. We shall consider now the rôle played by the spinal cord in conducting impulses to and from the brain. The fibers which enter the cord through the posterior roots of the spinal nerves bring in *afferent* impulses. Many of these impulses are carried upward by definite tracts that end eventually in the cortex of the cerebrum, cerebellum or other portions of the brain. On the other hand, many of the impulses originating in the brain are conducted downward into the cord (*efferent impulses*) to reach one or more of the anterior horn cells. The efferent impulses are carried to muscles by fibers which arise from anterior horn cells. These ascending and descending pathways form a large part of the entire structure of the spinal cord, and an understanding of their anatomical arrangement is of fundamental importance in neurological diagnosis.

The *fiber tracts of the spinal cord* are not scattered and intermingled at random, but, on the contrary, those fibers possessing a given function are grouped together in more or less definite bundles. These bundles, or fiber tracts, are present in the white matter of the cord and are, for the most part, composed of myelinated fibers.

We may classify the tracts grossly into ascending and descending. The ascending tracts are composed of fibers which conduct their impulses upward toward the higher parts of the cord or brain. They constitute the sensory or afferent pathways. The descending tracts conduct impulses from the brain downward to the anterior horn cells of the gray matter in the spinal cord. These are the motor pathways. There are other tracts and fibers which may be either ascending or descending, the impulses they convey serving to connect and link together the various segments of the cord (association tracts).

Ascending (sensory or afferent) Paths.—All fibers conveying sensory impulses from the skin of the limbs and trunk, from the muscles, bones and joints, and from the viscera and blood vessels enter the cord through the posterior roots of the spinal nerves. Not all sensory impulses are qualitatively the same. In the peripheral nerves, there is no grouping of fibers according to the quality of sensory impulses carried, but there is considerable evidence to merit the conclusion that each nerve fiber is capable of carrying only its own quality of sensation.

Certainly, the end-organs in the skin and mucous membranes are highly selective in the quality of sensory impulses which they initiate.

Once the sensory impulses enter the spinal cord, they are carried to fiber tracts. Each fiber tract conducts impulses of definite types. Thus, all sensory impulses of temperature and pain are conducted in the lateral spinothalamic tract. The exact arrangement of all of these sensory conduction pathways to the brain is still imperfectly understood, but our knowledge of the most important ones is sufficiently exact to be of great clinical importance.

The most important sensory pathways are those concerned with the conduction of impulses of the following types: 1. Pain and temperature; 2. light touch; 3. deep sensibility (proprioceptive); 4. tactile discrimination; 5. vibration.

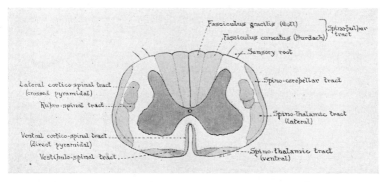

FIG. 29. Diagram of the spinal cord in cross section, indicating the location of the principal tracts.

1. Pain and Temperature.—All impulses of pain and temperature (heat and cold), whether cutaneous or deep, are carried to the posterior horns of gray matter, then to fibers which cross to the opposite side, within three spinal segments perhaps, ascend in the lateral spinothalamic tract and end in the thalamus (Fig. 29).

2. Light Touch.—Most of the impulses of light touch, after entering the cord, are carried to posterior horns of gray matter, then to fibers which cross to the opposite side, within several spinal segments, ascend in the ventral spinothalamic tract and end in the thalamus (Fig. 29). However, some impulses of light touch are carried upward by fibers in the posterior column of white matter of the same side. As a result of this double pathway, anesthesia to light touch is seldom produced by a lesion confined to one-half of the cord.

3. **Deep Sensibility (proprioceptive).**—Under this heading is included all sensibility mediated by afferent fibers from the muscles, tendons, ligaments, bones and joints. Deep sensibility proper is that ill-defined consciousness which we possess of the condition and position of our muscles, or of the joints or limbs moved by them. Most of these sensory impulses, certainly those which enter consciousness, are transmitted by the fibers forming the posterior columns (*fasciculus gracilis* and *fasciculus cuneatus*). These impulses enter the cord and ascend on the same side to the level of the medulla, where they end in the nucleus gracilis and nucleus cuneatus (Fig. 29). Other fibers conducting position sense undoubtedly end in the cerebellum. These fibers traverse the cord by way of the spinocerebellar tracts. The impulses thus transmitted furnish the afferent element in the reflex cerebellar control of muscular movement, particularly of the synergy necessary in locomotion.

4. **Tactile Discrimination (appreciation of two compass points when simultaneously applied).**—In the peripheral sensory distribution, tactile discrimination is closely allied to touch sensibility. However, in the cord, impulses of tactile discrimination are carried upward in the posterior column of white matter of the same side. Thus, when a lesion involves only the posterior columns, the sense of touch will not be affected, but tactile discrimination and deep sensibility will be lost.

5. **Vibration.**—Impulses of vibratory sense are transmitted upward in fibers which traverse the posterior column of white matter of the same side. Consequently, muscle sense, tactile

discrimination, and vibratory sense are usually abolished coincidentally, although one may suffer more than the other from incomplete lesions in this area of the cord.

It must not be inferred that the arrangement as described above accounts for all the afferent impulses which enter the cord. Many of them are "non-sensory" impulses which are concerned with the complex reflex mechanism which never reaches the level of consciousness (see chapter VI).

Descending (motor or efferent) Paths.—Fibers arising from cells in various parts of the brain descend in the spinal cord, forming several well-defined tracts. The most important of these motor tracts arise from cells in the motor cortex and continue down the cord as the corticospinal or pyramidal tracts (see p. 65). There are two of these pyramidal tracts on each side of the cord, the crossed and the direct. Only the crossed pyramidal tracts are of great clinical importance.

The Crossed Pyramidal Tract (lateral corticospinal).— The cells of origin of this tract lie in the motor cortex of the cerebral hemisphere. The fibers pass through the internal capsule and brain-stem to reach the spinal cord (Fig. 20). Just before they enter the spinal cord, they decussate in the medulla oblongata. After the decussation, the fibers assume a posterolateral position (Fig. 29). As the tract descends, it becomes smaller and smaller due to the distribution of fibers to cells in the gray matter of each segment.

The crossed pyramidal tracts, therefore, convey impulses from the motor portion of the cerebral cortex to the anterior horn cells. This represents the mechanism for the *voluntary* control of striated muscles. Moreover, the innervation is crossed; the right side of the brain controls the musculature on the left side of the body, and vice versa.

The *rubrospinal tract* is situated immediately ventral to the crossed pyramidal tract (Fig. 29). Its fibers arise from cells in the red nucleus and cross to the opposite side before entering the spinal cord to end in synaptic relation to anterior horn cells.

The red nucleus is intimately connected with every part of the cerebellum and corpus striatum. Destruction of it or severance of the rubrospinal tract causes marked disturbance in postural tonus. This tract is at least partly concerned with conduction of efferent impulses to the muscles of the body for the maintenance of muscle tonus.

The *vestibulospinal* tract is located in the anterior column of white matter (Fig. 29). Its cells of origin lie in the lateral nucleus of the vestibular nerve in the medulla oblongata. The fibers, after crossing in the medulla, terminate in synaptic relation to anterior horn cells. This tract conducts impulses concerned in the maintenance of body equilibrium.

Segmental Arrangement of Spinal Nerves

As indicated before, the spinal cord may be considered to be divided into segments. Each segment gives rise to a pair of spinal nerves. The component parts of each spinal nerve are a posterior and an anterior root. The spinal ganglion is located on the posterior root. The fibers of the anterior root (motor) have their cells of origin in the anterior horn of gray matter of the spinal cord. The posterior root fibers (sensory) arise from cells in the spinal ganglion. It is through this system of spinal nerves that the central nervous system is connected with the various end-organs in the periphery of the body (Fig. 28). A sharply defined segmental distribution of motor and sensory nerves is retained in the thoracic region in the adult, but distribution of fibers from other spinal nerves is complicated by the development of the limb buds during embryonic life. Opposite the attachment of the limb buds, the spinal nerves unite to form the brachial and lumbosacral plexuses. Each nerve which extends from these plexuses into the limb carries with it fibers from more than one spinal nerve. At first thought, such an intermingling of fibers would lead to hopeless confusion when attempting to determine the segmental distribution of sensory and motor fibers. As a matter of fact, the segmental arrangement can be recognized accurately even in the limbs, where the

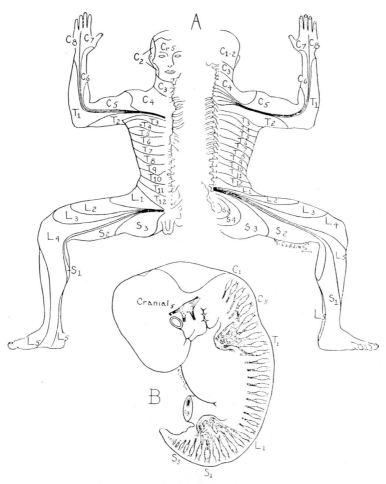

FIG. 30. Man as a segmental animal. A. Anterior and posterior views to show the sensory segmental distribution. B. The segments in the foetus, showing how the arms receive all the fibers of the brachial plexus, and how the legs receive those of the lumbar and sacral plexuses. (Homans)

distribution becomes most complicated (Fig. 30). It is through the knowledge of the segmental distribution of sensory and motor fibers that we are able to determine the exact location or level of a lesion in the spinal cord—hence, its importance to neurological diagnosis.

Sensory.—Corresponding to the spinal segments are areas of sensitivity upon the surface of the body. Perhaps the easiest way to remember the segmental sensory arrangement is to

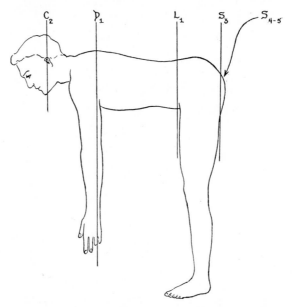

Fig. 31. Diagram of approximate sensory segmental distribution. "C," cervical; "D," dorsal (thoracic); "L," lumbar; "S," sacral.

project the body on all four extremities (Fig. 31). When this is done, the orderly distribution of sensory zones becomes apparent. The ulnar border of the upper limb corresponds to the first and second thoracic segments, the nipples to the fifth thoracic segment, and the umbilicus to the tenth thoracic segment. The front of the thigh corresponds to the lumbar segments and the back of the leg to the sacral segments. The perineal area corresponds to the fourth and fifth sacral segments.

Attention should again be called to the fact that the spinal cord segments do not correspond to the numerically corresponding vertebrae. For the relation between the spinal segments and the vertebral column see Fig. 32.

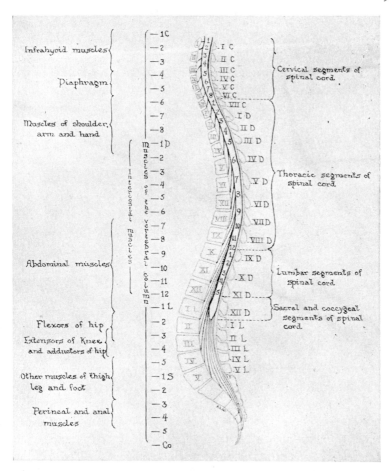

Fig. 32. Diagram showing the level of the various segments of the spinal cord with reference to the vertebrae. The table at the left of the drawing indicates the muscles innervated by the various anterior roots. (After Ranson)

Motor.—There is less evidence of segmental distribution of the motor fibers than of the sensory fibers. However, the fibers from the anterior roots are distributed in a very orderly manner. Only a few muscles are innervated from a single cord segment. The drawing in Fig. 32 indicates in a general way the segmental innervation of the voluntary muscles. Thus, if a muscle is innervated from a single anterior root, destruction of that root or segment of the cord from which it arises would cause complete paralysis of the muscle. If, however, the muscle is innervated from more than one cord segment, destruction of one motor root causes only weakness of the muscle. This explains the apparent irregularity in distribution and degree of paralysis seen in certain cases of poliomyelitis (infantile paralysis).

We may assume for sake of simplicity that the mechanism for voluntary control of muscles consists of two-unit chains, the upper motor neurons and the lower motor neurons. The *upper motor neurons* conduct impulses from the motor cortex to the anterior horn cells of the gray matter. From each anterior horn cell, a fiber passes out of the cord along the anterior root, enters into the formation of a peripheral nerve and ends at the motor end-plate in a muscle bundle. This lower segment of the motor path, which starts in the anterior horn of the cord and ends in the motor end-plate, is called the *lower motor neuron.*

A definite difference is observed in the paralysis caused by injury to the upper and to the lower motor neurons. Lesions of the lower motor neurons, whether they occur at the cell bodies in the anterior horn or in the peripheral nerves, cause paralysis, relaxation, and atrophy of the involved muscles (flaccid paralysis). The explanation of these phenomena is that the muscle is not only released from voluntary control but also from reflex activity, because the reflex arc is broken (see Chapter VI). Lesions of the upper motor neurons, whether they occur in the motor cortex of the cerebrum or at any point in the pyramidal pathways, cause paralysis from loss of voluntary control. Since the reflex arc is still intact, the muscles are still subject to reflex stimulation. Afferent impulses carried in, increase the tonicity of the muscles. Consequently, the muscles, after the stage of shock has subsided, are thrown into a state of hypertonicity in which they exhibit a spasticity (spastic paralysis).

As indicated in the discussion of the motor cortex, there has been some very substantial evidence presented which casts doubt upon the statement that spasticity is the product of upper motor neuron deficiency. The adherents to this newer conception maintain that lesions of the pyramidal system result invariably in flaccid paralysis, and that spasticity is purely a product of the extrapyramidal system, chiefly that part arising from the premotor area in the cerebral cortex. The evidence upon which this theory is based has been derived, for the most part, from animal experimentation. Its application to human cases has been largely a matter of conjecture.

Analysis of the paralytic phenomenon in the human, on the basis of the older view that spasticity results from pyramidal tract involvement, has been and continues to be very satisfactory in the vast majority of cases. The most difficult part of the phenomenon to explain is the temporary flaccidity which occurs as the result of acute lesions of the pyramidal system. Almost invariably, however, this stage is followed, after a period of weeks or even months, by spasticity. The newer theory of spasticity does not explain this change in tonicity any more satisfactorily than does the older one.

If we can think of the nervous system as being a closely knit and integrated whole instead of a series of isolated units, we will readily appreciate the fact that damage to any part will temporarily disturb the working smoothness of the entire system. The distribution of pyramidal fibers is profuse and probably embraces every reflex pathway involved in skeletal muscular activity. Sudden withdrawal of pyramidal activity in all probability temporarily "throws out of gear" all related reflex activity; then, after a period of time, the function of these reflex arcs is reëstablished. During the phase of reflex suppression, the paralyzed parts are flaccid. After the reflex arcs regain their activity, muscle tone returns, only at this time, it is without the "controlling" influence of the pyramidal system; hence, the incoming impulses elicit an exaggerated response, and a state of hypertonicity or spasticity results.

Visceral Innervation.—The nerve fibers which innervate the viscera and vascular systems, including all involuntary muscle and glandular tissue, possess certain distinguishing characteristics. The *efferent* fibers (preganglionic) are all finely myelinated, and their cell bodies for the most part lie in the intermediolateral cell column. These fibers leave the cord in the anterior root and pass to the ganglionated sympathetic trunk, or collateral ganglia, as white rami communicantes. Impulses are carried from cells in the sympathetic ganglia by postganglionic fibers to the involuntary muscles of the viscera and blood vessels and to the glands (Fig. 33). Many of these postganglionic fibers pass by way of the gray rami communicantes to the spinal nerves. Only those spinal nerves in the thoracic and lumbar regions possess both white and gray rami. Visceral *afferent* fibers take origin from unipolar cells in the spinal ganglia of the thoracic, upper lumbar, and sacral spinal nerves. The central processes terminate in the spinal cord. The peripheral processes run through the corresponding spinal nerves to the sympathetic trunk, through which they pass without inter-

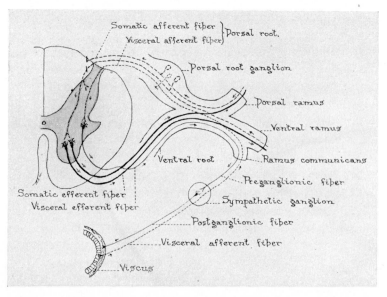

Fig. 33. Diagrammatic section through a spinal nerve and the spinal cord in the thoracic region to illustrate the chief functional types of peripheral nerve fibers. (After Ranson)

ruption in any of its ganglia. They may continue in the sympathetic system to end in the viscera, or they may again enter spinal nerves to end in the blood vessels. Thus, the smooth muscle of the viscera and blood vessels are supplied with a reflex mechanism through which afferent and efferent impulses may travel, and, for the most part, the reflexes thus initiated remain at a subconscious level.

CLINICAL.—In diagnosis of spinal cord lesions, it is not sufficient for the examiner to recognize that there is a lesion present which is producing certain abnormalities of function. He must, in addition, be able to determine the exact location of the lesion, not only with respect to the cord itself but to the vertebral column as well. In surgical diseases of the cord, exact localization of the lesion is of prime importance if the operative approach is to be planned and executed with precision.

The clinical examination of spinal cord function is conveniently divided into three parts: 1. Sensory system. 2. Motor system. 3. Reflexes. The discussion of the reflexes will be dealt with in a separate chapter (Chapter VI).

1. SENSORY SYSTEM

We have already considered the course and grouping of the chief sensory paths from the periphery to the brain. We have also discussed the segmental arrangement of superficial sensation and have pointed out the importance of this arrangement in the localization of spinal cord lesions. Let us now proceed to consider the methods of clinical examination of the various forms of sensation.

First of all, it should be remembered that the sensory examination is a subjective one, in that the observer is dependent upon the full coöperative accuracy of the patient in his response to the various tests. Care must be taken that the patient is not "tired out" before or during the course of the examination. It is a wise policy to delay the detailed sensory examination for a subsequent visit if he becomes fatigued or disinterested. In any event, no matter how perfect the setting for a satisfactory examination has been, the observations should be repeated one or more times in order to check their accuracy.

During the sensory examination, the patient should have his eyes closed or covered. He should not be asked leading questions as, "Is that sharp?" "Is that cold?" etc. An excellent code to use for the response to sensory stimuli is, "yes" for touch,

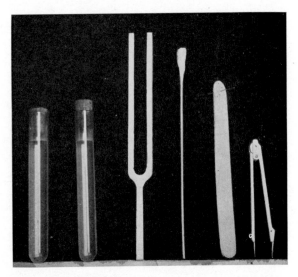

Fig. 34. Desirable equipment for the sensory examination.

"oh!" for pain, "hot" for a sense of heat and "cold" for a sense of cold.

No complicated apparatus is necessary to make accurate sensory tests. The desirable equipment is shown in Fig. 34.

The most important varieties of sensory stimuli which are generally employed in testing for sensory functions are light touch, pin pricks, hot and cold objects, point discrimination, passive movement of joints, and tuning-fork vibrations. The first four varieties of stimuli are tests for superficial (cutaneous) sensation, and the last two are tests for deep sensation. Each variety of sensation should be examined separately before passing on to the next kind of stimulus. No reliable conclusion can be drawn upon the sensory status until tests with every form of stimulus have been made. Thus, the sense of touch may be normal, yet pain and temperature sense may be lost. Or pain and temperature sensation may be normal and vibratory and joint sense absent. In mapping out areas of abnormal sensation, marks should be made on the patient's skin with a skin pencil—or more conveniently with a fountain pen—before recording the results on the sensory chart. When an area of diminished sensation is discovered, it is highly important to outline the margins of that area by working from the anesthetic area toward the normal skin, not in the reverse direction. It is far easier for the patient to recognize the exact moment when he feels a sensation than for him to observe when he first loses it.

The various forms of sensation are examined in the following order:

1. **Light Touch (tactile sensation).**—A small piece of cotton attached to a wooden applicator is a satisfactory instrument for testing perception of touch. If cotton is not available, a small pointed piece of paper serves very well. The skin is touched on a part relatively free of hair, and the patient is asked to indicate his first appreciation of the contact by saying, "yes." Corresponding areas of the two sides of the body are touched in sequence.

2. **Pain.** *A. Superficial pain.*—There is a wide variation in patients' responses to painful stimuli. A pin prick to one individual may be a very unpleasant sensation, while to another the same stimulus will produce only a mild discomfort. The examiner should always test the force of the stimulus on himself during the examination to be sure that a true unpleasant sensation is being produced, else he may not be actually testing for cutaneous pain.

An ordinary straight pin inserted through the end of a wooden tongue depressor or an open safety pin makes a very satisfactory tool for this test (Fig. 34).

Corresponding areas on the two sides of the body are tested alternately, care being taken to apply the same degree of pressure. There are, of course, minute spots in the skin where there are no pain end-organs; hence, a conclusion regarding pain sensibility cannot be reached by applying the pin point only once in a certain area, because of the likelihood of striking one of these spots. We are not only interested in demonstrating complete loss of pain sensibility (anesthesia), but also small degrees of pain loss (hypesthesia), as well as localized exaggeration of pain (hyperesthesia).

In case an abnormal pain area is suspected after a preliminary test of the whole body, it should be reëxamined most carefully with its boundaries marked out on the skin. In determining the boundaries of *hyperesthetic* areas, it is always better to work from the abnormal to the normal area. When a *hypesthetic* area is found, the reverse is true.

B. Deep pressure pain.—This variety of pain is examined by firm digital pressure applied to a muscle or its tendon. Pinching the tendon Achilles causes deep pain. Pressure on the testicle is another means of eliciting deep pain.

3. Temperature Sense.—This examination is made by means of two test tubes, one filled with hot water and the other with ice water, the outside of the tubes being thoroughly dried. If test tubes are not available, two metal objects of the same size (an ordinary teaspoon), one kept hot, the other cold by immersing in receptacles of water, make very satisfactory test objects.

Alternating hot and cold stimuli are applied on corresponding parts of the body. If there is a decrease in temperature sense more mistakes are likely to be made with the warm object than with the cold one. When there is complete loss of temperature sense, no difference is appreciated between the hot and cold objects.

4. Point Discrimination.—This test is best made by the simultaneous application of the two points of a compass to the skin, the distance between the points being varied until each point is felt separately. Normally, this distance is greater in the direction of the long axis of the body and smaller in the direc-

tion perpendicular to it. Normally, the distance between the two
points differs in the various parts of the body as follows:

Finger tips ....3 to 4 mm.
Back of hand ....30 mm.
Palm of hand .... 8 mm.
Forearm ....40 mm.
Arm and thigh ....80 mm.
Dorsum of foot ....40 mm.
Toes ....12 mm.

The patient is instructed to say "one" or "two" according to
whether he feels one or two points. The distance at which he
feels two points is recorded and compared with the normal for
the part being tested.

5. Joint Sense (sense of position).—Tests for this type
of sensation are made by moving a joint passively into various
positions, then holding it fixed in a certain position, and asking
the patient to imitate exactly the position with the limb of the
opposite side. He must, of course, keep the eyes closed, his
limbs relaxed, and refrain from voluntary motion of the limb
held by the examiner.

Another test is for the examiner to move the great toe, ankle,
thumb, or wrist into a position of extension or flexion and ask
the patient whether the part is pointing upward or downward.
This test is accurate only in cases with marked loss of joint
sensibility.

6. Vibratory Sense.—This test is made by means of a
medium pitched tuning-fork (C_256) which is set into vibration
and placed firmly on the styloid process of the radius and ulna,
the olecranon, clavicle, ilium, tibia and lateral and medial mal-
leoli. Normally, a distinct vibratory thrill is felt. This should
not be confused with the sense of touch or discomfort caused
by pressure of the fork upon the skin.

CLINICAL TYPES OF SENSORY DISTURBANCES

1. The Brown-Séquard Syndrome (lateral hemisection
of the cord).—This type of disturbance occurs most frequent-

ly from stab or gunshot wounds, but is not infrequently observed from spinal cord tumors. The syndrome consists of paralysis on the side of the lesion (spastic below the level and flaccid at the level of the lesion), loss of vibratory and position sense on the same side as the paralysis (due to destruction of the dorsal column which conveys position and vibratory sensation from the same side of the body), loss of pain and temperature on the opposite side of the body below the level of the lesion (due to destruction of the lateral spinothalamic tract which conveys the pain and temperature sensation from the opposite side of the body), and light touch acuity only slightly impaired on both sides below the level of the lesion (due to the fact that the fibers conveying touch sensibility ascend in the cord, partly in the ventral spinothalamic tract of the opposite side, and partly in the posterior column of the same side).

2. **Transverse Lesions of the Cord.**—This lesion results in the blocking (completely or incompletely) of all types of sensory impulses which enter the cord below it. Together with the sensory defects, spastic paralysis of the muscles below the level and flaccid paralysis at the level of the lesion are found. There are, in addition, sphincteric disturbances and pathological reflexes present. Transverse lesions result from compression of the cord by tumors, disease of the vertebrae, localized infection of the meninges, traumatic and vascular lesions of the cord and meninges. The degree of compression determines whether the lesion is complete or incomplete. With incomplete compression motor impairment with spasticity is often the first symptom. The posterior columns are the most sensitive of the sensory tracts to compression and the spinothalamic tracts the least sensitive. For these reasons pyramidal tract and posterior column signs often represent an early stage of spinal cord tumor and must not be too readily attributed to degenerative diseases of the cord.

3. **Syringomyelia.**—A lesion in the region of the central canal of the cord may, by expansion, destroy the pain and temperature fibers as they decussate in the anterior commissure on

their way to the lateral spinothalamic tracts. Such a lesion produces a loss of pain and temperature in this area without involvement of the other forms of sensation (touch and position sense). If the lesion grows sufficiently large, the other tracts of the cord will eventually become involved, and a transverse lesion will occur. Since the fibers conducting temperature appreciation lie on the mesial surface of the lateral spinothalamic tract, loss of this form of sensation below the level of the lesion may occur before the pain fibers become involved. Also, since the lesion involves the gray matter first of all, flaccid paralysis with atrophy of muscles supplied by these segments occurs early in the disease.

4. Tabetic Dissociation.—This lesion affects primarily the fibers which enter the dorsal columns of the cord, and, consequently, the disturbance produced is loss of vibratory and position sense with a preservation of pain, temperature and touch sensibility. This type of sensory disturbance may occur in other diseases than syphilis of the cord, notably, multiple sclerosis and pernicious anemia.

5. Hysterical Sensory Disturbances.—Functional sensory disturbances may *almost* simulate any known organic lesion. However, with careful sensory tests, one can usually demonstrate conclusively the difference between functional and organic lesions. In the first place, hysterical sensory loss is almost always complete, affecting all forms of sensation equally. In the second place, the sensory defects almost never conform to anatomical patterns of peripheral or central distribution. Characteristically, hysterical anesthesia involves a part equally anteriorly and posteriorly, with a sharp circumscribed line where the normal sensation suddenly appears, i.e., the "stocking" and "glove" anesthesias so frequently seen. The line of demarcation between the anesthetic and normal areas is usually sharply defined.

The anesthesia is often accompanied by motor paralysis, and in such cases, the organic signs of upper or lower motor neuron paralysis are invariably wanting.

2. Motor System

When any degree of muscular weakness exists, the patient, as a rule, recognizes it early and will so inform the examiner during the subjective examination. If the weakness affects the muscles of the upper extremities, the first complaint may be that he drops objects thought to have been firmly grasped, or he has difficulty in buttoning the clothing when dressing. If the lower extremities are involved, the patient usually complains of dragging the toes when walking, stumbling, or difficulty in ascending stairs. When the muscular weakness becomes more pronounced, his complaint may be that of "paralysis" of the involved parts.

The term "paralysis" should be defined. By *paralysis,* we mean a loss of voluntary motor power due to interruption, functional or organic, in any part of the motor pathway, from the cerebral cortex down to and including the muscle fibers. It is customary in some clinics to speak of *paralysis* as denoting a complete loss of voluntary motor power. Lesser degrees of impairment are then called *paresis.* General usage of the term *paralysis* to include partial as well as complete loss of power makes it desirable for us to use the term in its broader meaning, speaking, therefore, of *partial* or *total paralysis.*

Certain mechanical disturbances may be present in an extremity which will cause the patient erroneously to regard his loss of function as paralysis, notable among which are muscular or ligamentous strains, fractures, ankylosed joints, bursitis, or periostitis. Such conditions should be excluded before assuming that any degree of paralysis exists.

Paralysis may affect one extremity or any combination of extremities. When only one extremity is affected, the disturbance is called *monoplegia.* When one side of the body (face, arm, trunk and leg) is affected, the paralysis is spoken of as *hemiplegia.* When both legs, or both legs and trunk are paralyzed, the disturbance is called *paraplegia.*

We should begin the objective examination of the motor system by inspection of the limbs, noting the posture of each and the presence or absence of local muscular atrophy or hypertrophy. We should observe especially whether the muscles of the affected parts are rigid, stiff and spastic, or whether they are loose, relaxed and flaccid. We should then proceed to test the voluntary movements of the affected limb or limbs, always whenever possible using the normal member for comparison. It is not sufficient to ask the patient to move the arm or leg, as the case may be. Each joint should be tested separately, and all possible movements should be performed. Then the movements should be performed against resistance offered by the examiner—in case of the upper extremity, by elevating the arm when force is applied downward by the examiner, or in case of the lower extremity, by holding the limb against the examining table and making him elevate it against resistance. The simplest and most accurate test of strength in the upper extremities is for the patient to grip the examiner's fingers with both his hands simultaneously. Allowing for the handedness of the individual, the strength should be approximately the same on the two sides. When any degree of paralysis exists, the loss of strength in the affected hand will be easily demonstrated. To determine whether a particular muscle is taking part in a movement requires very close observation, not only by inspection but by palpation of the muscle or its tendon while the motion is being executed.

When paralysis exists, the affected muscles may be either normal in size and consistency, or enlarged and stronger than usual (*hypertrophy*), or diminished in size and strength (*atrophy*). In some cases, the muscles may be larger than normal but very weak, so-called *pseudohypertrophy*. This statement on first thought would appear to be paradoxical, but when we recall that organic paralysis may be caused by lesions at two different levels of the nervous system, upper motor neuron and lower motor neuron, and that the paralysis produced at each level shows usually certain distinguishing characteristics, then the variations observed in the paralyzed muscles themselves become more understandable.

For sake of emphasis, let us again define what we mean by

the upper and lower motor neurons. The portion of the voluntary motor tract from the cerebral motor cortex to the junction with the motor cells in the anterior horn of gray matter of the spinal cord is called the *upper motor neuron.* The motor pathway which starts with the anterior horn cell and continues in the peripheral nerve to end in the muscle fiber is called the *lower motor neuron.*

The distinguishing characteristics of lesions involving these two levels are shown in the following table:

ORGANIC MOTOR PARALYSIS*

Upper Motor Neuron	*Lower Motor Neuron*
1. Diffuse muscle groups affected, never individual muscles.	1. Individual muscles may be affected.
2. Spasticity or hypertonicity of paralyzed muscles.	2. Flaccidity or hypotonicity of paralyzed muscles.
3. Many have superadded "associated movements" on attempted voluntary movement.	3. No "associated movements."
4. No muscular atrophy except from disuse.	4. Atrophy of paralyzed muscles.
5. Electrical reactions normal.	5. Electrical reactions of degeneration.
6. Deep reflexes in paralyzed limbs present and usually increased.	6. Deep reflexes of paralyzed muscles diminished and often absent.
7. If foot affected, plantar reflex extensor in type.	7. Plantar reflex, if present, is of normal type.

* From Purves-Stewart.

The state of tonicity of paralyzed muscles is ordinarily the most accurate guide as to whether the lesion involves the upper or lower motor neurons. Spasticity or hypertonicity is characteristic of lesions of the upper motor neurons. This hypertonic state results from the release of the spinal reflex arcs from pyramidal control. In acute lesions, as for example, in apoplexy or cord injuries, it does not set in immediately. There is an initial period of flaccidity gradually replaced after a few days or weeks by spasticity, the so-called "late rigidity." When the onset of the paralysis is more gradual, as for example, in a tumor involving the corticospinal pathways, the paralysis is spastic from the beginning. The degree of spasticity may be estimated fairly accurately by passively moving the patient's joints, and comparing the resistance offered to such movements with that of the healthy limb.

The differential diagnosis between an upper and lower motor neuron lesion is, as a rule, simple. While no one sign listed in the table is infallible when considered singly, yet the sum of the seven signs enables one to determine with great accuracy which neuron is involved in any given case. It must not be forgotten that not infrequently one may encounter paralysis which is due to a combination of upper and lower motor neuron lesions. For instance, with a tumor involving the last four cervical spinal cord segments, the arms would present the characteristic findings of lower motor neuron paralysis, due to destruction of the anterior horns and anterior roots in the affected segments, while the rest of the body below the arms would be involved in a spastic paralysis from interruption of the pyramidal tracts.

Urinary Bladder Disturbances in Lesions of the Cord.— Vesical control is not purely a motor phenomenon, but since it is accomplished normally through a voluntary motor act, we shall consider it at this point.

Like most of the internal organs of the body, the urinary bladder has a double innervation: 1. From the second to the fifth lumbar nerves, efferent fibers reach the bladder through the sympathetic chain. 2. From the second and third sacral spinal nerves, efferent fibers take their course through the nervi erigentes and the hypogastric plexus. These two sets of nerves are antagonists. Thus, stimulation of the sacral nerves causes strong contraction of the bladder with relaxation of the internal sphincter, while stimulation of the lumbar sympathetics causes acceleration of tone in the sphincter and inhibition of contraction of the bladder musculature.

The sensory nerves from the bladder pass through the sacral autonomics by the rami communicantes and along the posterior roots to the spinal cord. In normal circumstances, the desire to urinate undoubtedly results from a pressure stimulation of the sensory fibers from accumulation of urine in the bladder.

Micturition in the adult is a voluntary act, but only to the extent that it can be voluntarily initiated. The first step in the act is accomplished by contracting the abdominal walls and fixing the diaphragm, thus raising the intravesical tension. Next, the voluntary striated constrictor muscle of the urethra is relaxed, while the involuntary non-striated internal sphincter is inhibited. The rise in intravesical pressure starts the reflex by which the smooth muscle of the bladder wall contracts. Once started the bladder empties itself spontaneously, and the only way that the act can be stopped is by compression of the voluntary constrictor of the urethra, usually a matter of considerable effort.

In the course of almost every disease of the spinal cord, bladder disturbances are eventually encountered. Usually, the disturbance is due to an involvement of the nervous mechanism by which the patient loses voluntary control of micturition. In acute transverse lesions of the cord, especially when both motor and sensory pathways are involved, a complete retention of urine is encountered, as, for example, in traumatic injury to the vertebral column with cord compression. At first, the bladder becomes over-distended and atonic with little or no effort on the part of the bladder musculature to overcome the tonic contraction of the internal sphincter. After a certain stage of over-distention occurs, the intravesical tension becomes sufficiently high to cause an "overflow" dribbling in which the excess urine runs away continuously through the urethra without the bladder musculature making the necessary effort to overcome the distention of its walls. Needless to say, frequent catheterization, or better still, an "indwelling" catheter is of great importance in the prevention and treatment of over-distention of this sort.

After a few days, particularly if the bladder has not been allowed to become tremendously over-distended, the bladder musculature will begin to regain its contractile power, and while the voluntary mechanism for micturition is still lost, the bladder wall will regain sufficient tone to eliminate a large "residual urine," which would otherwise be drawn off only by gravity through the catheter.

After several weeks or months following such a spinal cord injury, the stage of initial retention comes to an end. By this time, the contraction of the bladder musculature has become sufficiently vigorous to overcome the tonic activity of the internal sphincter, so that catheterization may no longer be required. Any stimulation, for instance pinching of the thigh, may be sufficient to initiate the reflex for emptying the bladder completely. This is the *reflex* or *automatic* bladder.

In spinal cord lesions of more gradual onset, bladder disturbances usually appear late in the course of the disease. For instance, in tumors and degenerative lesions of the spinal cord, months or even years may elapse during which time the patient may become severely incapacitated from motor or sensory impairment before vesical disturbances are noted. However, if the lesion is confined to the sacral segments of the cord, urinary symptoms may be the first to appear. If the lesion involves parts of the cord above the sacral segments, retention of urine is the rule. If it be confined to the sacral segments, incontinence or dribbling of urine is most frequently noted.

The patient with spinal cord disease may deny any urinary difficulties except that an additional effort is required to start the act of micturition. Yet, when the abdomen is examined, a distended bladder reaching to the umbilicus may be found. Such a patient, while able to void certain quantities of urine voluntarily, maintains a high residual urine due to the fact that he is able to reduce the intravesical pressure only to a certain point beyond which he has no voluntary control. When such a bladder is examined with the cystoscope, marked hypertrophy of the muscle bundles offers ample evidence of the effort the organ has made to complete the emptying process.

LOCALIZATION OF SPINAL CORD LESIONS

Many diseases of the spinal cord affect from the beginning one or more parts of the cord throughout its entire length.

Therefore, in this type of case, the exact level at which normal function leaves off and abnormal function begins is of little or no clinical importance. However, it is most important for purposes of differential diagnosis to recognize accurately just what functional units of the cord are involved. For instance, in tabes, the posterior columns and dorsal roots are involved first, while in primary lateral sclerosis, the crossed pyramidal tracts are involved almost exclusively.

There are many diseases of the cord which are sharply localized to one, two or three segments (tumors, abscesses, syringomyelic cavities, vascular lesions, compression from traumatic injuries to the spine, caries of the spine, etc.). In these types of lesions, accurate knowledge of the exact level, not only with respect to the cord itself but the vertebral column as well, is important. If the treatment is surgical, then such accurate localization becomes essential. If there is no specific treatment to be offered, then an accurate localization is a reward for diagnostic acumen.

It is entirely due to the segmental arrangement of the spinal cord that we are able to locate precisely, from clinical examination, the exact level of a given lesion. Such a clinical examination consists of obtaining information with regard to: 1. Sensory level. 2. Sympathetic level. 3. Motor level.

1. **Sensory Level.**—By utilizing the tests for the various forms of sensation as described in the preceding pages, one may determine with great accuracy the level where normal sensation ceases and abnormal sensation begins. It must be constantly borne in mind that a sensory examination utilizing one form of stimulus, for instance, pin prick, is not sufficient to determine the sensory status. After the sensory level or line has been obtained and marked on the patient's skin, then a sensory chart should be consulted and the level marked upon this chart, indicating the quality of sensory changes that occurs at each level (Figs. 35, 36). This level indicates the segment of spinal cord where the upper level of the lesion lies, and this level may

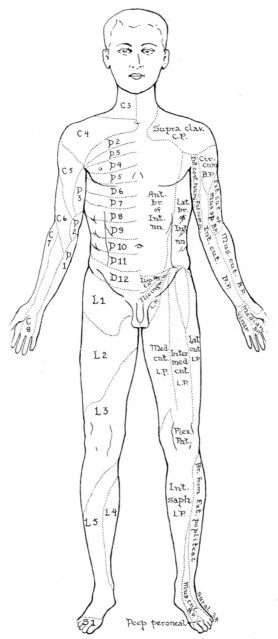

Fig. 35. Segmental sensory chart (anterior view). The sensory segmental
zones are shown on the left half of the body; the sensory distribution of
the peripheral nerves is shown on the right half of the body.

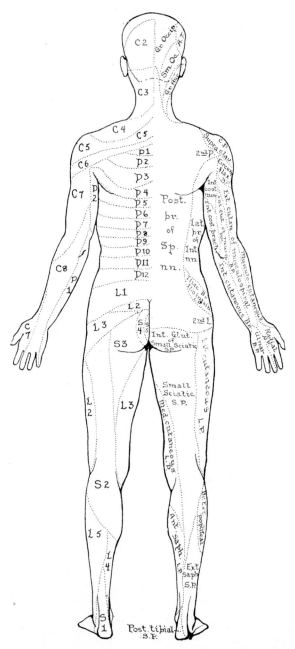

Fig. 36. Segmental sensory chart (posterior view). The sensory segmental zones are shown on the left half of the body; the sensory distribution of the peripheral nerves is shown on the right half of the body.

be located in regard to the vertebral column by consulting Fig.
32. It will also be noted that in mapping out areas of abnormal
sensation on the chart, one may ascertain at a glance whether
such areas correspond to segmental or peripheral nerve distribution. Not infrequently, in spinal cord tumors, the posterior
roots at the level are pressed upon sufficiently to cause severe
radiating pains. When root pains occur, one may map out the
distribution very accurately and this, of course, may be one of
the most valuable means of determining the exact level of the
lesion.

2. **Sympathetic Level.**—The activity of the sweat glands
is controlled by sympathetic nerves. Overactivity of these
nerves produces an excess of sweat, underactivity a decrease or
disappearance of sweating. Transverse lesions of the spinal
cord are associated with abnormalities of sweating due to involvement of cells in the intermediolateral column of the gray
matter. Below the level of the lesion, the skin is dry; above this
level, the skin is moist. This sweat line can be easily demonstrated by gently passing the finger tips over the surface of
the skin from below upward, and when the area of normal
sweating is encountered, there will be a distinct "pull" or
"hang" on the finger tips. The line demonstrated in this manner
usually coincides closely with the sensory level.

This test can be demonstrated more clearly following administration of pilocarpin. Profuse sweating is produced in the
parts above the level of the lesion, whereas the skin below the
level will remain dry.

3. **Motor Level.**—As has been pointed out previously, the
segmental arrangement of the motor nerves is much more complicated than is the sensory system. This is due to the fact that
individual muscles are usually innervated from more than one
cord segment, so that involvement of the motor fibers from one
does not completely destroy function.

The following table indicates the approximate segmental distribution of the motor roots of the spinal cord:

C^4	Posterior group of neck muscles.
C^5	Deltoid, biceps, brachialis anticus, supinator longus.
C^6	Pronators of the forearm.
C^7	Triceps, extensors of the wrist and fingers.
C^8	Extensors of the wrist and fingers.
Th^1	Small muscles of the hand.
Th^{2-10}	Intercostal muscles.
Th^{7-12}	Muscles of the abdominal wall.
$TH^{12}-L^3$	Psoas.
L^3	Adductors of the thigh.
L^4	Quadriceps, abductors of the thigh.
L^5	Hamstrings.
S^1	Glutei, posterior calf muscles.
S^2	Anterior tibials, peronei, small muscles of the foot.

CHAPTER VI

THE REFLEXES

In the previous chapter, we have considered the spinal cord as a pathway for the conduction of impulses to and from the brain. We shall now consider this organ from the standpoint of its reflex activity. The spinal cord, on the one hand, acts simply as a connecting link between the brain and the peripheral nervous system, and, on the other hand, it becomes an organ independent, to a degree, of its connections with the brain. This independence is due to its extensive series of reflex centers through which control of the activities of the viscera, blood vessels, numerous glands, and, to some extent, the entire voluntary muscular system is mediated.

ANATOMY AND PHYSIOLOGY.—The functional unit of all reflex activity is the reflex arc. This arc may be simple or complex, but regardless of its complexity, it always consists of the following parts:

(a) The afferent or inward path which is composed of a receptor organ (sensory ending) connected to an afferent nerve fiber. The afferent nerve fiber enters the spinal cord by the posterior root.

(b) The reflex center in the central nervous system.

(c) The efferent or outward path composed of efferent nerve fiber and end-organs. The efferent fiber leaves the spinal cord by way of the anterior root.

The reflex arc in its simplest theoretical form is composed of a two-neuron chain. The *afferent* or *sensory neuron,* after entering the cord through the posterior root, ends, after profuse branching, on the cell body of the *efferent* or *motor neuron* in the anterior horn. The secondary neuron consists of the motor nerve cell and its processes, the peripheral process of which leaves the spinal cord by the anterior root to end at an end-organ in the muscle or gland (Fig. 37). The reflex act, which results from a stimulus passing over this simple reflex arc, occurs in the following manner: The sensory nerve ending (receptor), having received a stimulus sufficiently great to produce a nerve impulse, transmits it to the spinal cord by way of the afferent fiber in the posterior root. After entering the cord, the impulse is transmitted through the synapse of the afferent neuron to the efferent (motor) cell. The impulse is

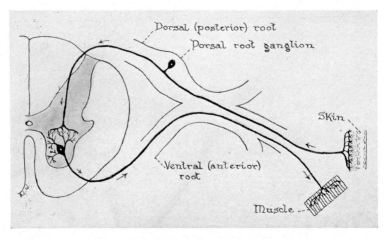

Fig. 37. Diagram of the simple reflex arc.

then carried away from the cord by the efferent fiber where it is transmitted to the muscle fibers through the motor end-plate. As a result of this impulse, there is contraction of the muscle fibers which shortens the muscle and a movement results.

A simple reflex is probably a purely abstract conception. All parts of the nervous system are intimately connected, and no part of it is ever capable of reacting without affecting and being affected by various other parts. However, from the standpoint of simplicity and understanding, it is helpful to analyze complex reflexes and reduce them as nearly as possible to their simple components.

Probably the nearest approach we have to an example of a simple two-neuron reflex arc is the *tendon reflex*. As the most familiar example, let us consider the knee-jerk, and try to explain the mechanism by which it is produced. When the patel-

lar tendon, as it passes over the knee-joint, is tapped with a
reflex hammer, a number of tension receptors are subjected to a
very sudden stretch. The vol-
ley of impulses thus initiated
is carried to the spinal cord
over the afferent fibers. Upon entering the cord, these
impulses pass through a
series of branching collaterals of the afferent fibers,
through intermediate neu-
rons to the motor cells of the
anterior horn, and thus ex-
cite a series of motor impulses which leave the cord
over the efferent fibers to end
in the motor end-organs of
the quadriceps extensor muscle. The sudden contraction
of the quadriceps muscle
constitutes the knee-jerk.

The more complex re-
flex acts are accomplished
through a mechanism which
provides for connections between the various segments
on the same and opposite
sides of the cord, the medulla and brain. While the
anatomical connections for
such reflex actions are many
and varied, the following description of a complex reflex
pathway will serve as an example of spinal reflex activity.

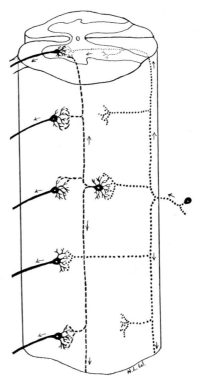

Fig. 38. Diagram illustrating the
mechanism of a diffuse unilateral reflex.
...... Afferent (sensory) neuron
which, after entering the cord, divides into ascending and descending
branches.
- - - - - Intermediate (association)
neuron.
———— Efferent (motor) neurons.

Almost immediately after entering the cord, the afferent fiber
splits into two main branches. One branch passes downward,

the other upward in the cord, and collaterals from these main branches may be given off to each segment in passing (Fig. 38). The course pursued by these branches is of variable length. Many of the ascending branches reach the brain, but the others terminate, as do the descending branches and all the collaterals, in the gray matter of the cord. In the gray matter, these branching afferent fibers connect with intermediate or association neurons which in turn connect with the primary motor neurons. Through this system of association fibers, connections are made with the various segments on the same side of the cord to produce *unilateral reflexes*. Other fibers cross the cord in the white or gray matter to end at the primary motor neurons of the opposite side, thus providing a mechanism for *crossed reflexes*.

According to this conception of reflex pathways, one sensory fiber may establish connections directly or indirectly with a great number of motor cells on the same or opposite side of the cord, or with the brain. In this manner, a sensory fiber carrying an impulse which eventually reaches the cerebral cortex, thus giving rise to a conscious sensation, may, by means of its collaterals, connect with motor cells in the cord and medulla, thereby producing at the same time involuntary or subconscious reflexes.

As an example of a reflex of this kind, let us suppose that the finger tip has been suddenly brought into contact with a lighted match. By the time one is conscious of the pain, the muscles of the whole upper extremity have contracted, and perhaps the entire body has been moved a step backward to increase the distance between the finger and the source of the painful stimulus. At the same time, there has occurred a reflex stimulation of the vasomotor center, resulting in constriction of the small arteries of the finger. Thus, this original stimulus to the pain and temperature receptors of the finger has spread over this network of afferent collateral fibers and association neurons to the brain, medulla, and many segments of the spinal cord to effect a purposeful reflex action.

The importance of reflex activity in maintaining the body in its daily environment should be obvious. All of our involuntary acts and the basis for many of our voluntary acts are reflex in nature. For instance, walking, singing, dancing, and even automobile driving, although in the beginning effected by voluntary coördination, nevertheless in the end become more or less entirely reflex actions. All voluntary acts, if deprived of their reflex components, would assume grotesque forms. Thus, in the voluntary movement of the limb, the movement is guided and "smoothed out" by reflex activity which maintains muscle tonus and keeps an even balance between antagonistic groups of muscles.

Inhibition of Reflexes.—A fundamental characteristic of spinal reflexes is the fact that they can be inhibited by other impulses reaching the same part of the spinal cord, i.e., they can be depressed or suppressed entirely. For instance, we know that by a voluntary act we can temporarily inhibit respiratory movements or the act of micturition, both of which are normally under reflex control. Likewise, it is possible by voluntary effort to inhibit the reflex which would normally occur after pricking or tickling the sole of the foot. A similar inhibition of reflex activity may be obtained by the simultaneous stimulation of two different parts. For instance, by firm pressure upon the upper lip, the reflex of sneezing can often be completely inhibited.

Use of Spinal Reflexes as Diagnostic Signs

The knee-jerk is perhaps the most widely used of the spinal reflexes in clinical diagnosis. This, like all other tendon reflexes, depends upon the integrity of the reflex arcs in the spinal cord. Any disease which breaks any part of the arc will abolish it. In tabes, for instance, the posterior root fibers in the lumbar cord are affected, and, as a consequence, the reflex is diminished or abolished, according to the stage of the disease. So, also, lesions affecting the anterior horn cells or roots, poliomyelitis as an example, will destroy the reflex by interrupting the motor path. Lesions affecting the corticospinal system, anywhere from the motor cortex to the pyramidal tracts of the cord, are accompanied by exaggeration of this and similar reflexes. This phenomenon is due to the removal of the inhibitory influences of the brain centers which act, normally, upon the spinal reflex mechanism.

Almost any tendon if stimulated mechanically will give a jerk of the corresponding muscle. It is often important in clinical diagnosis to establish a *level* at which the disease process begins or ends. In such circumstances, the condition of the tendon reflexes may be of valuable aid, particularly if the tendon reflex arcs through successive levels of the cord are utilized. Thus, the tendon reflexes of the upper extremity test the reflex arcs from the fifth cervical to the second thoracic segments. The reflexes of the lower extremity test the integrity of the pathways from the second lumbar to the third sacral segments.

A second group of spinal reflexes offers valuable aid in neurological diagnosis—the superficial or cutaneous reflexes. This group consists of the abdominal, cremasteric and plantar reflexes. The first two, abdominal and cremasteric, are abolished by any disease which destroys or depresses the reflex arcs from the tenth thoracic to the second lumbar segments. Unlike the tendon reflexes, disease of the pyramidal tracts causes diminution or disappearance of these reflexes. The plantar reflex consists normally of plantar flexion of the toes when a tactile or painful stimulus is applied to the sole of the foot. When the pyramidal tracts are diseased, this normal reflex is altered so that the great toe is extended (dorsiflexed)—the Babinski phenomenon.

CLINICAL.—We are concerned clinically with *superficial* and *deep* reflexes. The superficial reflexes are obtained by gently stroking or scratching the skin with some blunt object. The deep reflexes are obtained by brisk percussion of the tendon of a muscle with a soft rounded object, preferably a rubber reflex hammer.

Superficial Reflexes.—Several of the superficial reflexes have already been described in connection with the examination of the cranial nerves. They are the corneal (p. 42), the ciliospinal (p. 38), and the pharyngeal (p. 54) reflexes. The other important ones are the abdominal, cremasteric and plantar reflexes.

Abdominal Reflexes.—These reflexes can best be elicited with the patient recumbent. The abdominal walls must be relaxed. The skin of the abdomen is stroked with a blunt point, preferably a match or a wooden applicator. In testing for the upper abdominal reflex, the skin of the right and left upper abdominal quadrants is stroked. This causes contraction of the muscles of the upper abdominal wall, thus producing deviation of the umbilicus to the side of the stimulus. The lower abdominal reflex is obtained by stroking the skin of the lower abdominal quadrants. The muscles of the lower abdominal walls contract and thus pull the umbilicus outward and downward.

The pathway for the upper abdominal reflex is through the ninth and tenth thoracic segments. For the lower abdominal reflex, the pathway is through the eleventh and twelfth thoracic segments.

These reflexes are frequently absent in elderly people, in multiparae, and the very obese patients. Any healed lateral abdominal incision may cause them to disappear on the side of the incision, due to the disturbance by the scar of the neural pathways. In acute peritoneal inflammation, they may disappear completely.

Cremasteric Reflex.—Pricking or stroking the skin of the inner side of the thigh causes contraction of the cremasteric muscle, thus lifting the testicle on that side. This reflex varies considerably in normal individuals; hence, it may be an unreliable sign unless it coincides with the other clinical findings. The arc concerned in this reflex is through the first lumbar segment.

Plantar Reflex.—The normal plantar reflex consists of plantar flexion of the toes, especially the great toe, when the outer side of the sole of the foot is stroked from the heel forward (Fig. 39). A blunt point (the end of a match or toothpick) should be used to produce this response. The stimulus should be made firmly and slowly. Some patients are so sensitive on the sole that it is impossible to employ the test because of the defense reaction. In such circumstances, the test should be tried

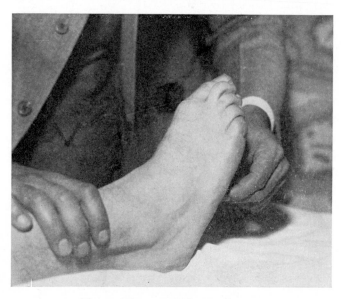

Fig. 39. The normal plantar response.

with the knee flexed and the leg resting across the opposite knee. In this manner, the defense reaction is reduced considerably.

The reflex pathway of the plantar response is through the first and second sacral segments.

In pyramidal tract lesions, an extensor (dorsiflexion) movement of the great toe with spreading, or "fanning" of the other toes occurs. This phenomenon is called the sign of Babinski (Fig. 40).

This reaction is a sign pathognomonic of pyramidal tract involvement except in two conditions. The first is in infants up to the age of 10 or 11 months in which a dorsiflexion of the great toe is normal. The second exception is in those cases of lower motor neuron paralysis (e.g., poliomyelitis) in which the only intact muscles in the foot are the extensors of the toes, and, consequently, the only response possible to a plantar stimulus is one of dorsiflexion. The *Babinski sign,* aside from the two exceptions given above, *is always pathognomonic of organic disease of the pyramidal tracts.*

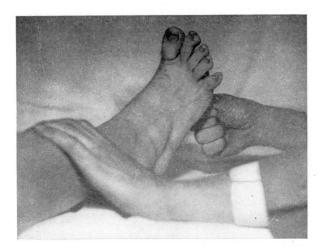

Fig. 40. The Babinski reflex.

When the Babinski sign is doubtful, there are a number of tests which are of considerable corroborative value.

The *Oppenheim sign* consists of dorsiflexion of the great toe in response to firm stroking from above downward of the inner border of the tibia.

The *Gordon sign* consists of dorsiflexion of the great toe when the calf muscles are firmly grasped and squeezed.

The *Chaddock sign* consists of dorsiflexion of the great toe after stroking beneath the lateral malleolus and along the dorsum of the fifth metatarsal. This confirmatory sign is very valuable because it eliminates the "tickling" reaction.

Not infrequently, in severe pyramidal tract lesions, all of these plantar reflexes are present. Occasionally, a positive response can be elicited by the simultaneous application of the Babinski and Gordon tests.

All of the superficial reflexes are dependent upon cerebral reflex arcs as well as spinal reflex arcs for their completion. Therefore, if either component of the spinal arc is broken, the reflex is abolished. For instance, if the skin is anesthetic because of a central or peripheral lesion, the superficial reflex for this area is not obtained. Likewise, if the motor component is affected,

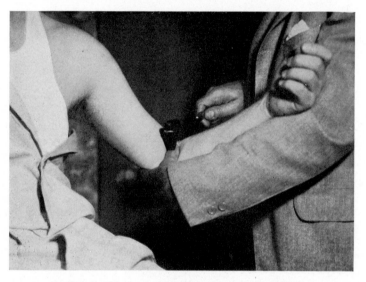

Fig. 41. Method of obtaining the biceps reflex.

the reflex is absent. If the cerebral pathway is broken by disease of the pyramidal tract above the segment of the cord controlling the motor response, the reflex is abolished.

Considerable evidence of localizing value may be obtained by study of the superficial reflexes. If, for example, the upper abdominal reflexes are intact, and the lower abdominals and the cremasterics are lost, we have presumptive evidence that the upper level of the lesion is at the eleventh or twelfth thoracic segments.

Deep Reflexes.—The deep reflexes consist of the tendon and periosteal reflexes. Except in rare instances, they are present in all normal individuals and are equal on the two sides of the body.

The following reflexes are commonly tested:

1. The Biceps Reflex is best obtained by resting the relaxed forearm of the patient on the left arm of the examiner (Fig. 41). The examiner's left thumb is placed on the biceps tendon, and the tendon stimulated by striking the thumb a sharp blow with the reflex hammer. The biceps muscle is seen to contract, and the patient's forearm flexes slightly as a result of the contraction. The arc is through the fifth and sixth cervical segments.

2. The Triceps Reflex is obtained by placing the forearm of the patient in the same position as for the biceps-jerk (Fig. 42). The tendon of the triceps is struck directly with the reflex hammer near its insertion at the olecranon process. The muscle is seen to contract, and a slight extension of the forearm results. The arc is through the sixth and seventh cervical segments.

3. The Radial Periosteal Reflex (supinator) is not a true

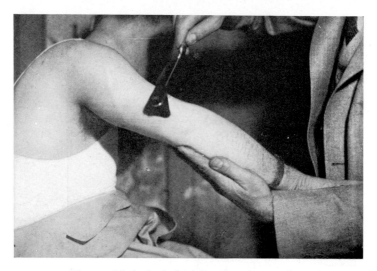

Fig. 42. Method of obtaining the triceps reflex.

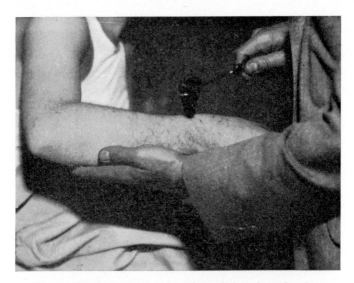

Fig. 43. Method of obtaining the radial periosteal reflex.

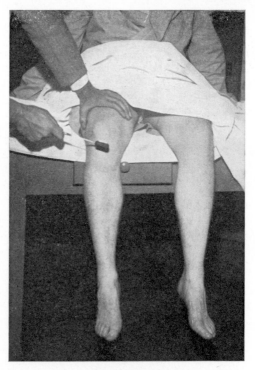

Fig. 44. Method of obtaining the knee-jerk with the patient seated.

tendon reflex. It is obtained in essentially the same position as used for the biceps and triceps reflexes (Fig. 43). The styloid process of the radius is struck briskly with the reflex hammer. The response elicited consists of a slight flexion of the fore-arm and often a slight flexion of the fingers and the wrist. The reflex pathway is through the seventh and eighth cervical segments.

4. **The Knee-Jerk.**—There are many ways in which this reflex can be elicited, depending upon whether the patient is

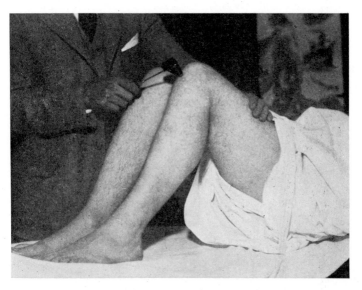

FIG. 45. Method of obtaining the knee-jerk with the patient recumbent.

seated or recumbent. When the patient is seated, the legs should hang loosely over the edge of the examining table or chair so that the feet do not touch the floor (Fig. 44). The tendon of the quadriceps extensor is struck just below the patella. A brisk contraction of the muscle normally results in a "kick" of the leg. It is desirable for the examiner to place the left hand on the quadriceps muscle so that he may feel the contraction, and thus a better comparison of the two sides is possible. Not infrequently, a contraction can be felt when there is not sufficient force to cause extension of the leg.

When the patient is recumbent, the knees should be bent in such a manner that the soles of the feet rest flat against the table (Fig. 45). Contraction of the quadriceps resulting from a blow on its tendon causes an extension of the leg with a movement forward of the foot which rests on the table. In this position, it is particularly important to palpate the contraction in the muscle, so that the amount of force on the two sides can be estimated.

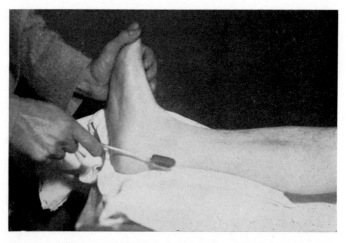

FIG. 46. Method of obtaining the ankle-jerk.

Not infrequently, this reflex is difficult to elicit, due to the patient's inability to relax the limb. A most useful maneuver consists of "locking" the hands together and pulling either constantly or in jerks just previous to the tapping of the tendon. This, or a similar voluntary effort, results in *reënforcement* of the knee-jerk.

The arc for the knee-jerk is through the third and fourth lumbar segments.

5. **The Ankle-Jerk (Achilles' jerk)** is obtained by placing the foot at a right angle to the leg with gentle traction exerted

on the "ball" of the foot by the left hand of the examiner (Fig. 46). Tapping the tendon of Achilles causes a brisk contraction of the gastrocnemius and soleus muscles, thus resulting in plantar flexion of the foot. Relaxation must be complete. Any voluntary contraction of the anterior tibial muscle will completely inhibit the ankle-jerk. A useful maneuver for securing complete relaxation is to have the patient kneel on a chair grasping the back of the chair firmly with the hands. The examiner then applies slight pressure to the "ball" of the foot and strikes the Achilles' tendon a brisk blow. If no reflex response is obtained in this position one may feel assured that the Achilles' jerk is absent. The pathway is through the first and second sacral segments.

6. Ankle-Clonus.—When the foot is quickly and forcibly pushed up into extreme dorsiflexion and held there by moderate pressure, a clonic contraction of the gastrocnemius and soleus muscles may result, thus producing an oscillation of the foot (Fig. 47). The phenomenon is called ankle-clonus and represents nothing more than a series of exaggerated ankle-jerks,

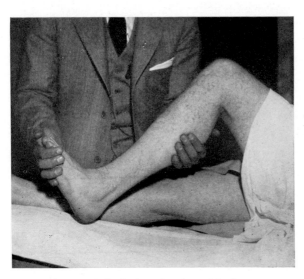

Fig. 47. Method of testing for ankle-clonus.

elicited in a different way. These movements may be either *transient* or *sustained*, depending upon the degree of hyperactivity. Ankle-clonus is not invariably a sign of organic disease, as it may occur in highly nervous individuals after prolonged illnesses or after severe muscular exertion. But when it is combined with reflex inequalities or other signs of organic disease of the cord, it is a most significant finding.

Pathological States in Which the Deep Reflexes Are Diminished

1. In diseases of the joints (acute and chronic), muscles (myopathies) and tendons (traumatic), the deep reflexes in that region may be diminished or absent.

2. After prolonged administration of sedative drugs (bromide, phenobarbital, etc.), the deep reflexes may be greatly diminished.

3. In lesions of the peripheral nerves, such as toxic neuritis from alcohol or lead, inflammatory lesions like sciatic neuritis, and traumatic injuries to the nerves, the regional deep reflexes are diminished or absent.

4. In lesions of the dorsal columns of the cord, such as tabes and combined sclerosis, the deep reflexes are diminished or absent, due to the break in the afferent side of the reflex arc.

5. In lesions of the anterior horn cells, such as poliomyelitis, syringomyelia, and primary muscular atrophy, the deep reflexes are abolished, due to the break in the efferent side of the reflex arc.

6. In acute injuries to the cord involving the pyramidal tracts, these reflexes are, as a rule, abolished for a time, varying from a few weeks to months. Usually, the state of diminished reflex activity is followed by a great exaggeration of the deep reflexes.

Pathological States in Which the Deep Reflexes Are Increased

1. In the neuroses and psychoneuroses, the tendon and periosteal reflexes are, as a rule, exaggerated. This hyperac-

tivity is not accompanied by other signs of organic disease of the pyramidal tracts, such as abolition of the superficial reflexes and the presence of a positive Babinski reaction.

2. In a lesion of any sort involving the corticospinal pathways, whether it be in the motor cortex, internal capsule, pons, medulla or spinal cord, there is an exaggeration of the deep reflexes below the level of the lesion on the side to which these fibers are ultimately distributed. In amyotrophic lateral sclerosis an unusual situation exists. In addition to anterior horn degeneration, as in primary muscular atrophy, there is degeneration of the corticospinal system. For this reason hyperactive reflexes are often observed even in the presence of muscular atrophy. The only exception to this rule is in the case of acute injuries to this system; in which case, the reflexes may be temporarily abolished.

3. In tetanus and strychnin poisoning, the deep reflexes may be exaggerated.

CHAPTER VII

SUMMARY AND CLINICAL IMPRESSION

After the examination has been completed and the details recorded in the order indicated in the outline, all of the positive findings should be summarized, briefly and concisely. It is desirable, for the sake of clarity, to separate the subjective from the objective findings. When this is done, one may procure, by glancing through the *summary,* the salient facts elicited by the history and the neurological examination. If more detailed information regarding any particular point is desired, reference may then be made to that section of the record dealing with the point in question. A record thus summarized is of great convenience to the examiner and consultants, in that all the positive data are brought together and a minimum of effort is required to review the pertinent details of the case.

One should always attempt to record a clinical impression after the neurological examination is completed. In a large percentage of cases, the clinical impression will consist of a differential diagnosis, the final diagnosis being delayed until, through subsequent examination and a consideration of the data accumulated from laboratory tests, more information becomes available. In some cases, it is impossible to arrive at a positive diagnosis even with the help of all available data. In such instances, the passage of time may so clarify the clinical picture as to make an accurate diagnosis possible.

REFERENCES

1. BRAIN, W. R., and STRAUSS, E. B., *Recent Advances in Neurology,* Second Edition, P. Blakiston's Son & Co., Inc., Philadelphia, 1930.
2. DANA, C. L., *Textbook of Nervous Diseases,* Ninth Edition, Wm. Wood & Co., New York, 1923.
3. FORD, F. R., *Diseases of the Nervous System in Infancy, Childhood and Adolescence,* Charles C Thomas, Springfield, 1937.
4. FULTON, J. F., "Personal Communications."
5. FULTON, J. F., JACOBSEN, C. F., and KINNARD, M. A., "A Note Concerning the Relation of the Frontal Lobes to Posture and Forced Grasping in Monkeys," *Brain,* 55, 4, 1932.

6. GRAY, H., *Anatomy of the Human Body,* Twentieth Edition, Lea & Febiger, Philadelphia, 1931.
7. HERRICK, C. J., *An Introduction to Neurology,* Fifth Edition, W. B Saunders Co., Philadelphia, 1931.
8. HOLT, E., and McINTOSH, R., *Diseases of Infancy and Childhood,* D. Appleton & Co., New York, 1933.
9. HOWELL, W. H., *A Textbook of Physiology,* Twelfth Edition, W. B. Saunders Co., Philadelphia, 1933.
10. MAY, C. H., *Manual of the Diseases of the Eye,* Thirteenth Edition, Wm. Wood & Co., New York, 1930.
11. McKENDREE, C. A., *Neurological Examination,* W. B. Saunders Co., Philadelphia, 1928.
12. McNEILL, CLYDE, *Roentgen Technique,* Charles C Thomas, Springfield, 1939.
13. MONRAD-KROHN, G. H., *The Clinical Examination of the Nervous System,* Second Edition, H. K. Lewis & Co., Ltd., London, 1923.
14. PURVES-STEWART, SIR JAMES, *The Diagnosis of Nervous Diseases,* Sixth Edition, E. B. Treat & Co., New York, 1924.
15. RANSON, S. W., *The Anatomy of the Nervous System,* Fourth Edition, W. B. Saunders Co., Philadelphia, 1931.
16. SHERRINGTON, C. S., *The Integrative Action of the Nervous System,* Yale University, New Haven, 1906.
17. TILNEY, F., and RILEY, H. A., *The Form and Functions of the Central Nervous System,* Second Edition, Paul B. Hoeber, Inc., New York, 1923.
18. WECHSLER, I. S., *A Textbook of Clinical Neurology,* W. B. Saunders Co., Philadelphia, 1930.
19. WRIGHT, S., *Applied Physiology,* Fourth Edition, Oxford University Press, London, 1921.

PART II

THE CEREBROSPINAL FLUID

CHAPTER VIII

THE CEREBROSPINAL FLUID

The examination of the cerebrospinal fluid has become such an important step in neurological diagnosis that it is essential for the student to have a clear understanding of the anatomy of the cerebrospinal fluid spaces, and the condition of the fluid in health and disease. Moreover, there are so many clinical disorders in which the symptomatology is almost entirely dependent upon a disturbance of the normal circulation of the fluid, that this knowledge is doubly important.

ANATOMY AND PHYSIOLOGY

The cerebrospinal fluid spaces may be divided, for sake of clarity, into an *internal* and an *external* system. The internal system is composed of the two lateral ventricles, a relatively

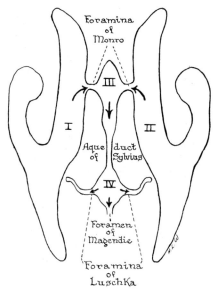

FIG. 48. Diagram of the ventricular system of the brain to show the circulation of the cerebrospinal fluid: I, II, the lateral ventricles; III, the third ventricle; IV, the fourth ventricle. The arrows show the direction of flow of the cerebrospinal fluid. (Modified from Howell)

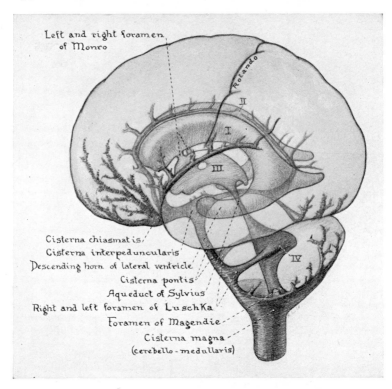

Fig. 49. Diagram of the cerebrospinal fluid spaces: I, II, the lateral ventricles; III, the third ventricle; IV, the fourth ventricle. The other important landmarks are labelled. (After Dandy)

small third ventricle lying between the cerebral hemispheres, and the fourth ventricle in the medulla oblongata. The third and fourth ventricles are connected with each other by a slender canal traversing the midbrain, called the aqueduct of Sylvius (cerebral aqueduct) (Fig. 48). The central canal of the spinal cord properly belongs to this internal system as it connects above with the fourth ventricle, and contains cerebrospinal fluid. However, this structure in man is so rudimentary that it is seldom considered to be a part of the cerebrospinal fluid pathways.

The external system is composed of the subarachnoid spaces lying over the surfaces of the brain and spinal cord, the large dilated subarachnoid cisternae, and the perivascular and peri-neural extensions of the subarachnoid space which surround the blood vessels of the brain and the cranial and spinal nerves (Fig. 49).

Communication between the internal and external systems is established through an opening in the roof of the fourth ventricle (foramen of Magendie) and the two lateral openings in the lateral recesses of the fourth ventricle (foramina of Luschka) Fig. 48. These three openings provide the only means of communication between the ventricular system and the sub-arachnoid spaces. Moreover, they are very tiny openings, being difficult to identify with the naked eye. The continued patency of these foramina is essential for the normal circulation of the cerebrospinal fluid. Thus, closure from disease results in *internal hydrocephalus*—a condition which, if complete, is in the adult incompatible with life.

The ventricular system is lined by a thin membrane called the ependyma, the inner layer of which is composed of ciliated epithelium. The large lateral ventricles are separated from each other by the *septum pellucidum,* but communicate with the third ventricle and indirectly with each other through the inter-ventricular foramina (foramina of Monro).

The choroid plexus lies on the floor of the lateral ventricles. It is composed of tiny blood vessels arising from the choroidal arteries. The veins of the plexus empty into the internal cere-bral veins. The plexus is covered by a layer of epithelium which is a continuation of the ependymal lining of the ventricle. Thus, the choroid plexus projects into the ventricular cavity but does not actually lie in it because of the continuation of the epithelial lining of the ventricle over its surface. This struc-ture in its relationship to the ventricular cavity is identical to the projection of the intestinal tract into the abdominal cavity. The tufts of the choroid plexus are largest in the lateral ven-tricles. The extensions of the plexus pass through the foramina of Monro into the third ventricle. There is also a tuft of choroid plexus in the roof of the fourth ventricle but it is a separate unit.

The external or subarachnoid system is formed by the space lying between the inner two meningeal layers which cover the brain and spinal cord. The meningeal layers from without inward are termed *dura, arachnoid* and *pia*.

The dura consists of tough fibrous tissue lined by endothelium. In the skull, it splits into an outer and an inner layer. The outer layer forms the endosteal lining of the cranial bones, and the inner layer (cerebral dura) envelops the brain. The outer layer ceases at the foramen magnum of the skull; the spinal dura is a continuation of the cerebral dura.

Separating the dura from the arachnoid is the subdural space containing a small amount of clear fluid. Under normal conditions this space is in no way connected with the cerebrospinal fluid pathways. Moreover, there is no absorptive mechanism present in the subdural space, an anatomical defect of great clinical importance because of the frequency in which blood is extravasated into this space as a result of head injuries. Blood thus extravasated acts as a foreign body, becomes encapsulated by proliferation of the endothelium from the inner layer of dura and, because of the absence of an absorptive mechanism, lies latent in the subdural space, gradually giving rise to the condition known clinically as *subdural hematoma*.

The arachnoid is separated from the pia by a space of varying size called the *subarachnoid space* which contains the cerebrospinal fluid. The pia is closely adherent to the nervous substance and dips into all the fissures of the brain and spinal cord. The arachnoid does not follow the pia into the fissures but invests the whole nervous system quite loosely. At several points, the subarachnoid space becomes tremendously dilated, thus forming the *cisternae*. The most important of the cisternae are: (1) the cisterna magna, found between the medulla and the under surface of the cerebellum; (2) the cisterna pontis, lying on the anterior aspect of the pons; (3) the cisterna chiasmatica, lying about the optic chiasm, above the pituitary body; (4) the cisterna interpeduncularis (basilar cistern) formed by the arachnoid bridging across the space between the tips of the temporal lobes (Fig. 49).

Prolongations of the subarachnoid space extend along the sheaths of the cranial and spinal nerves. Also, as the arteries and veins enter and leave the brain substance they are invested by the perivascular spaces which are continuous with the subarachnoid space.

Thus, every part of the central nervous tissue is in contact directly or indirectly with the cerebrospinal fluid.

Formation.—The chief source of the cerebrospinal fluid is the choroid plexus. Perhaps a part of the fluid is formed in the perivascular spaces and in the ependymal lining of the ventricles, but these sources represent an insignificant part of the total amount of fluid produced. The rapidity with which the fluid is formed under normal conditions is still a moot question. When the lateral ventricle is opened at the operating table and the choroid plexus brought into direct vision, one may observe the formation of fluid. After first sponging the plexus dry with cotton pledgets, within a couple of minutes, a small pool of newly formed fluid is observed. This observation may be repeated again and again with the same result. Certainly, if under normal conditions of intracranial tension fluid were formed at this rate, the total volume (110-130 c.c.) would be changed every 3 to 4 hours. It is generally estimated that the total volume of fluid is changed every 6 to 8 hours.

The formation of cerebrospinal fluid may be satisfactorily explained as a process of filtration through a membrane of characteristic permeability. The semipermeable membrane is probably made up of the capillary endothelium and the layer of epithelial cells which covers the plexus. Many of the constituents of the blood plasma are present in the cerebrospinal fluid in about the same proportions. Any significant change in the concentration of glucose, sodium chloride, and urea in the blood stream is at once reflected in the fluid. On the other hand, all colloidal substances and certain inorganic substances like sodium iodid and sodium nitrate are held back and do not appear in the fluid even when highly concentrated in the blood stream. In deep jaundice, for instance, while all other bodily fluids are stained, the cerebrospinal fluid remains relatively clear. There is no doubt, therefore, that the cells of the choroid plexus exert some selective activity over the substances which are allowed to diffuse into the cerebrospinal fluid.

Absorption.—Most of the fluid is absorbed into the dural venous sinuses by means of the arachnoidal villi which project

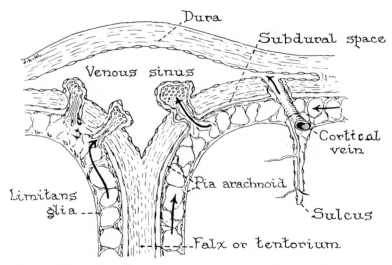

FIG. 50. Diagram to show relations of pia-arachnoid, the arachnoid villi, and cortical veins to the dural sinuses. (Cushing-Weed)

into them. A small part of it may pass into the blood stream directly by way of the perivascular spaces (Fig. 50). Also, a part of the fluid which covers the spinal cord may be absorbed into the spinal veins.

The pacchionian bodies (arachnoidal granulations) are large collections of arachnoidal villi present for the most part along the superior longitudinal sinus. They are not present in infancy and are rarely found until after the third year. As they grow, they cause absorption of bone from pressure and so produce the pits or depressions in the inner table of the skull in the vicinity of the longitudinal sinus. These bodies, for many years, have been considered to be the important if not the only mechanism for the absorption of cerebrospinal fluid. Weed has shown conclusively that there are innumerable arachnoidal villi projecting into the venous sinuses, large and small, cortical and basilar (Fig. 50). He believes that these villi are the most important absorptive pathways, and that the rôle of the pacchionian bodies has been greatly exaggerated.

Dandy goes a step further and claims that cerebrospinal fluid is absorbed from every part of the subarachnoid space through the capillary walls, just as other body fluids are absorbed. Be that as it may, it is sufficient for our purposes to understand that the fluid is absorbed into the blood stream through some mechanism lying in the subarachnoid system, and that little or none of it is absorbed in the ventricular system. Therefore, for the newly formed fluid to be disposed of properly, it must escape from the ventricular into the subarachnoid system.

Circulation.—The cerebrospinal fluid is constantly circulating in the sense that it is being continuously secreted and absorbed. The fluid formed by the choroid plexus of the lateral ventricles passes through the foramina of Monro into the third ventricle and thence through the aqueduct of Sylvius into the fourth ventricle. Its mode of exit from the fourth ventricle is by way of the medially placed foramen of Magendie and the two laterally placed foramina of Luschka whence it enters the large cisterna magna of the subarachnoid space. From the cisterna magna, the fluid passes in two directions: (1) upward and forward about the base of the brain to reach the surface of the cerebral hemispheres; (2) downward in the spinal subarachnoid space over the surface of the spinal cord. Thus, the cerebrospinal fluid is in continuous movement, in a definite direction through a highly specialized pathway.

Functions.—The cerebrospinal fluid has at least three important functions: 1. It serves as a medium for the transfer of substances from the tissues of the brain and spinal cord to the blood stream. 2. It serves as a space compensating mechanism in regulating the contents of the cranium. 3. It serves as a fluid buffer against injury.

The first of these functions, the medium of exchange of substances from the tissues of the brain to the blood stream, is perhaps the most important. Examination of normal fluid from different loci of the nervous system, i.e., the ventricle, cisterna magna, and the spinal subarachnoid space, discloses the fact that the further away from the choroid plexus one obtains the specimen of fluid, the higher its nitrogenous content. For instance, from the cerebral ventricles, the total protein content is about 10 mgm. per 100 c.c., from the cisterna magna about 20 mgm. per 100 c.c., and from the spinal subarachnoid space about 40 mgm. per 100 c.c. Presumably, this increase in protein content represents the end-product of metabolism which is constantly being discharged into the cerebrospinal fluid for ultimate disposal in the blood stream. On the other hand, there is no reliable evidence that the fluid carries nutritive material from the blood stream to the nervous tissue, inasmuch as the sugar and chloride contents of the fluid do not change significantly in the different loci. In this respect, the cerebrospinal fluid resembles lymph.

That the cerebrospinal fluid acts as a medium of exchange for secretions from the posterior lobe of the pituitary body, and perhaps the pineal gland, is probable, although difficult to prove. Cushing has offered evidence to support the belief that pituitrin is constantly being discharged into the cerebrospinal fluid, and through its presence in the fluid, some control over the vasomotor and heat centers in the hypothalamic region is effected.

The second of these functions, the space compensating mechanism, is undoubtedly of great importance. The brain is enclosed in a rigid and inexpansible chamber after childhood, and any marked change in the volume of the brain must be immediately adjusted, or else intracranial pressure variations would be tremendous. Rapid space compensation is possible only through the medium of fluid. The only two fluid substances normally in the brain are blood and cerebrospinal fluid.

Sudden change in intracranial volume is probably compensated for chiefly by variations in volume of the vascular bed.

The vessels of the brain are supplied with vasomotor fibers, so the quantity of arterial blood distributed to the various parts of the brain substance may be changed minute by minute with the same rapidity as occurs in any organ of the body.

More gradual changes in intracranial volume are probably accomplished through an increase or decrease of cerebrospinal fluid. For instance, in lesions attended by a loss of brain substance such as occurs following trauma, infection, or arterial occlusions, enlargement of the contiguous ventricle and subarachnoid space compensates for this loss. In expanding lesions of the brain such as neoplasms, abscesses, or hemorrhages, there is a reduction in the size, or even obliteration of the contiguous fluid reservoirs with an actual decrease in the volume of cerebrospinal fluid.

The third function of the cerebrospinal fluid is that it acts as a fluid buffer against injury. This conception is believed by many to be more theoretical than real, particularly in case of the brain. However, the large dilated cisternae, lying between the hypothalamic regions, pons, and medulla, and skull unquestionably offer some protection from trauma to these very vital parts of the brain. In the spinal cord, the fluid-filled subarachnoid space surrounding the cord must offer considerable protection.

Composition.—Under normal conditions, the cerebrospinal fluid is clear, colorless, and slightly alkaline in reaction. Its specific gravity is 1.004 to 1.006. It consists chiefly of water and contains the inorganic salts of the blood plasma in about the same concentration. Its protein content varies from 0.01 to 0.04 per cent and consists of albumin and globulin. The dextrose content varies between 0.05 and 0.08 per cent. A few cells resembling lymphocytes are found. Their number does not exceed 5 per cu. mm. and usually is from 1 to 2 per cu. mm.

CLINICAL

LUMBAR PUNCTURE.—Samples of cerebrospinal fluid may be obtained for analysis by puncture of any part of the fluid confines. Three sites are in common usage: 1. Lateral ventricles. 2. Cisterna magna. 3. Lumbar subarachnoid space.

The first two sites, the cerebral lateral ventricles and cisterna magna are available only to those who through training and experience have acquired the necessary technical skill to make the procedures safe. Puncture of the lumbar subarachnoid space (lumbar puncture), on the other hand, is a procedure which, if properly understood, especially as to the indications and contraindications, is almost as safe as puncture of a vein. Also, if performed skillfully, the patient experiences little or no discomfort. However, no physician is justified in making lumbar puncture studies unless he is thoroughly familiar with the contraindications and unless he is equipped to recognize the physical signs upon which these contraindications are based.

Contraindications to Lumbar Puncture.—There are two contraindications to lumbar puncture which may be accepted as absolute:

1. A high degree of papilloedema (choked disc) from any cause.

2. Neurological evidence of an expanding lesion in the posterior fossa of the skull, with or without papilloedema.

1. *Choked discs* are almost always due to a high degree of intracranial pressure. The source of this increased pressure may be due to many causes, but, as a rule, it results from either a tumor or abscess increasing the bulk of the cranial contents by size alone, or from blockage of the free circulation of the cerebrospinal fluid thereby producing internal hydrocephalus. The latter condition may result from tumor, abscess, or inflammatory adhesions. Acute irritative or inflammatory lesions of the meninges characteristically produce a high degree of intracranial pressure, but ordinarily there is no blockage of the cerebrospinal fluid circulation associated with them. Also, acute lesions rarely produce choked discs. We may assume, therefore, that choked discs are the product of increased intracranial pressure which has existed for sometime, and that the lesion producing this pressure is either a space-occupying one or one

which blocks the exit of the cerebrospinal fluid from the ventricular system of the brain.

We should recall again that the cranial contents are separated into two compartments by the tentorium cerebelli, the only connections between the two being at the incisura of the tentorium through which the midbrain passes (p. 89). The *supratentorial* chamber houses the cerebral hemispheres, basal ganglia, and the hypothalamus. The *subtentorial* chamber houses the cerebellum, pons, and medulla.

An expanding lesion of the cerebral hemispheres causes a general increase of intracranial pressure, but the tension is greater in the *supratentorial* fossa. Likewise, obstruction of the third ventricle blocks the exit of fluid from the lateral ventricles and thereby produces internal hydrocephalus. Again the pressure above the tentorium is greater than that below it.

If, in such circumstances, fluid is suddenly withdrawn by lumbar puncture, the subtentorial pressure is acutely reduced, but the greater supratentorial pressure is at first unaffected. This inequality of pressures predisposes to further herniation of that part of the midbrain normally lying above the tentorium into the incisura, thereby strangulating it. At the same time, the great veins of Galen, which empty into the dural venous sinuses, may be compressed or strangulated, thereby causing a degree of venous stasis incompatible with life.

These facts probably explain satisfactorily many of the sudden deaths which have occurred following lumbar puncture in the presence of supratentorial tumors.

2. Lesions lying below the tentorium produce at first the greatest increase of pressure in the *subtentorial fossa*. It is only after the fluid exits from the fourth ventricle have been interfered with that a general swelling of the optic disc is to be expected.

The contents of the subtentorial fossa communicate with the spinal canal through the foramen magnum of the skull. Into the opening of the foramen magnum projects the medulla oblongata at the level of which it is continuous with the cervical spinal cord. As pressure in the posterior fossa increases, pressure in the spinal canal likewise increases as long as there remains free communication between the two. If the lesion be an expanding one, more and more of the cerebellum, which is the least fixed part of the brain in this chamber, becomes compressed into the aperture of the foramen magnum. If this herniation of cerebellar substance becomes sufficiently great, all of the brain substance in the foramen magnum, including the medulla, becomes strangulated and medullary failure supervenes.

If lumbar puncture is performed when this mechanism is still compensated, the sudden shift of pressure in the spinal canal predisposes to further herniation of cerebellar tissue, thereby hastening the strangulation. It is small wonder that

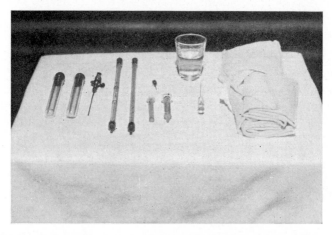

FIG. 51. Instruments and supplies used in lumbar puncture. From left to right: two test tubes with cork stoppers; lumbar puncture needle; spinal fluid manometers; hypodermic needle and syringe (2 c.c.); glass of 70% alcohol; ampule of 1% novocain; sterile towels and sponges.

sudden deaths following lumbar puncture in these circumstances are of all-too-common occurrence.

With these explanatory data in mind, it becomes obvious why a careful neurological study of every patient should precede lumbar puncture, whether it be done for purposes of diagnosis, or treatment. If, for any reason, examination of the cerebrospinal fluid appears to be necessary when these contraindications to lumbar puncture exist, the fluid can be much more safely obtained from the lateral ventricle, even though a small trephined opening in the skull is necessary.

Technique of Lumbar Puncture.—The first step in the preparation of a patient for lumbar puncture is complete reassurance as to the harmlessness and painlessness of the procedure. It should always be done in the patient's bed with just as little "fuss" in preparation as possible.

All of the necessary instruments and supplies for lumbar puncture are shown in Fig. 51.

The patient is brought to the edge of the bed and placed in a

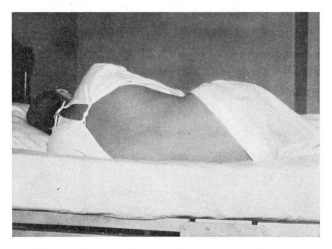

FIG. 52. First step in the lumbar puncture technique:
Position of the patient.

position in which the transverse axis of the body is perpendicular to the surface of the mattress (Fig. 52). He is then asked to "draw the knees up until they touch the abdomen and to bend the neck forward until the chin touches the chest." These movements automatically arch the vertebral column and separate the spinous processes. The head should be placed on the same level as the spinal column so that an accurate reading of the intracranial pressure can be made. Next, the crest of the

ilium is palpated with the fingers of the left hand and the left
thumb is placed on the spinous process which lies just above a

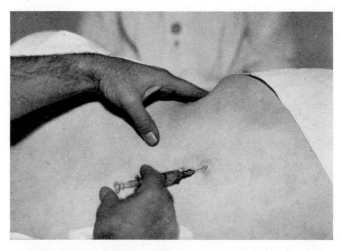

FIG. 53. Second step in the lumbar puncture technique: Novocainization of
the skin and soft tissues.

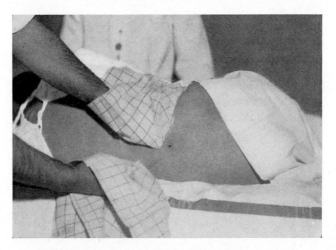

FIG. 54. Third step in the lumbar puncture technique: The sterile towel
technique for identification of the spinous processes and handling of the
spinal puncture needle.

line connecting the two iliac crests. This landmark usually
identifies the spinous process of the third lumbar vertebra. Then

the entire field is thoroughly cleansed with 70 per cent alcohol—or iodine and alcohol if one prefers. A wheal of one per cent procain is raised in the skin, exactly in the midline just below the spinous process of the third lumbar vertebra (Fig. 53). Then the remainder of the 2 c.c. syringe of procain is distributed just below the fascia in and to either side of the midline. Again, the field is cleansed with alcohol. Next, the operator places a sterile towel over the back in such a way that the left hand may be applied over it, so that the fingers are in contact with the iliac crest and the thumb palpates the third lumbar spinous process. With the right hand, he unfolds another sterile towel and picks up the lumbar puncture needle in the towel (Fig. 54). The needle is then inserted into the skin at the

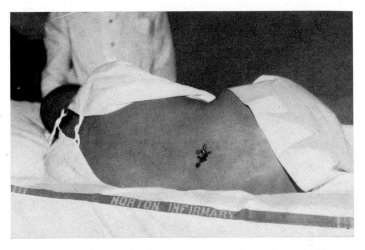

FIG. 55. Fourth step in the lumbar puncture technique: Needle inserted and stylet partially withdrawn.

anesthetized point just below the third spinous process; the left hand in position helps to identify this point. It is then inserted directly inward, attempting to remain in the midline at all times. At a depth of about 5 cm. in an adult of normal size, an increased resistance is felt as the needle pierces the ligaments between the laminae. If the point of the needle encounters bone, withdraw the needle about 2 cm. and direct the point slightly upward. As soon as this resistance of the ligaments is no longer felt, the stylet should be withdrawn from the needle with the "toweled hand," for not infrequently the needle has penetrated the dura and arachnoid without any sensation of "feel" on the part of the examiner (Fig. 55). If a drop of fluid is recovered from the needle, the stylet should be reinserted and preparations made for the application of the manometer. If fluid is not recovered, the needle should be pushed forward, millimeter by millimeter, until the subarachnoid space is entered.

At this point, the towels may be discarded and any further manipulation at the end of the needle may be made with a sterile gauze sponge.

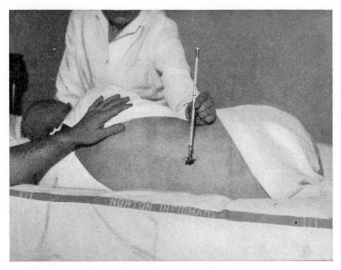

Fig. 56. Fifth step in the lumbar puncture technique: Manometer attached to needle preparatory to manometric readings.

Next, the manometer is applied to the needle and the pressure observed over a period of several minutes, while the patient is completely relaxed and breathing normally through his mouth (Fig. 56). Unless the patient is thoroughly relaxed, pressure readings will be higher than normal, because any mental agitation or physical tension raises the intracranial pressure.

After the dynamics of the cerebrospinal fluid have been studied, samples of the fluid are taken slowly—not more than 1 or 2 c.c. at a time—until sufficient fluid is obtained to carry out the necessary laboratory tests. Usually, 8 c.c. will suffice for a complete spinal fluid study.

The needle is then withdrawn quickly, and the puncture hole in the skin is cleansed with alcohol. If there is bleeding from the skin, pressure is applied until it ceases. No dressing of any sort is applied to the skin.

This lumbar puncture technique is simple, unpretentious, and flawless as regards asepsis, if properly performed. It can be carried out as conveniently in the patient's home as in the hospital. It eliminates the elaborate "set-up" for which some physicians carry the patient to the operating room.

The use of general anesthetics for lumbar puncture is not only rarely necessary, but makes an accurate measurement of the intracranial pressure impossible. All inhalation anesthetics raise intracranial pressure by producing venous congestion of the brain; hence, manometric readings under anesthesia are always higher than normal. If the patient is extremely apprehensive or delirious, one of the sedative drugs may be used as preliminary medication. Such drugs do not affect greatly the intracranial pressure.

CEREBROSPINAL FLUID DYNAMICS.—Since all of the cerebrospinal fluid spaces are, under normal conditions, in free communication, measurement of the pressure in one part will reflect the degree of tension in all other parts. For instance, if the pressure in the lumbar subarachnoid space is found to be 150 mm. of cerebrospinal fluid (water pressure), we may assume that the reading of 150 mm. reflects accurately the amount of pressure within the cranial cavity, *provided* there is no obstruction to the flow of fluid from the intracranial cavity to the lumbar subarachnoid space. Furthermore, if for any cause the intracranial tension should be raised temporarily, the change in pressure would be immediately transmitted to the lumbar subarachnoid space with a corresponding rise in the manometric reading.

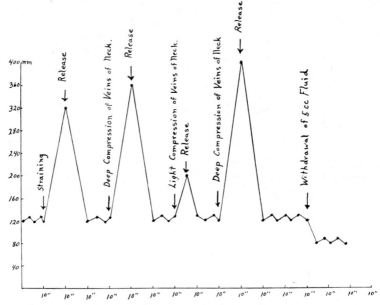

FIG. 57. Normal manometric chart showing respiratory and pulse oscillations, the prompt rise and fall on straining, light and deep jugular compression.

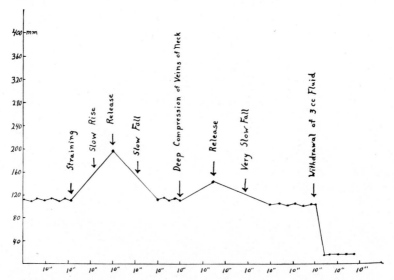

FIG. 58. Manometric chart showing complete subarachnoid block. Note the rise in pressure on straining is greater than from deep compression of the veins of the neck.

It is upon these data that the *Queckenstedt test* (jugular compression test) is based. When the internal jugular veins are compressed completely, the venous return from the intracranial contents is arrested; therefore, if the arterial supply continues to function, there occurs immediately a tremendous venous engorgement which in turn produces a great increase in intra-cranial pressure. If only one jugular vein is compressed at a time, venous congestion occurs but is moderate in degree. Also, if both jugular veins are only partially occluded the degree of venous congestion will depend upon the amount of impediment to venous return. The amount of intracranial pressure is always in direct proportion to the degree of venous congestion.

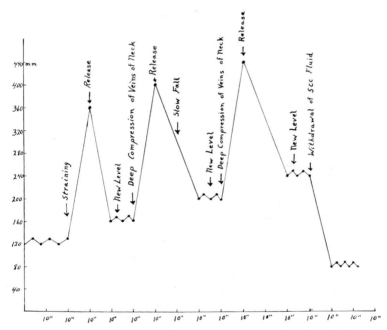

FIG. 59. Manometric chart showing incomplete subarachnoid block. Note the new pressure level after each test. Also the prompt rise and slow fall which occur after deep compression of the veins of the neck.

If the subarachnoid space from the level of the cisterna magna to the point of lumbar puncture is freely open and com-municating, all of these quick changes of intracranial pressure will be reflected immediately in the pressure of the lumbar fluid. As the venous stasis from jugular compression is increasing, the lumbar fluid will rise in the manometer. The moment the jugular pressure is removed and venous return is established, the fluid column will fall promptly until the normal level of intracranial pressure is established (Fig. 57). By noting the readings in millimeters on the manometer, a record of these changes of intracranial pressure may be recorded.

If an obstruction occurs in the spinal subarachnoid space at any point between the cisterna magna above and the point at which the lumbar puncture needle is inserted below, these changes in intracranial pressure cannot be transmitted promptly to the fluid column in the lumbar puncture manometer. If the obstruction is *complete,* no rise of pressure will be observed when the jugular veins are occluded (Fig. 58). If the obstruction is *incomplete,* a very slow rise will occur with deep compression, and a very slow fall of the fluid column will be observed after the compression is removed (Fig. 59). Furthermore, the initial pressure of the lumbar fluid is reduced very rapidly in complete or nearly complete obstructions with the withdrawal of a few drops of fluid, due to the fact that it is impossible or difficult to replace the withdrawn fluid from the supply above the obstruction. Coughing, straining, sneezing, or holding the breath in the inspiratory position will produce a rise in the lumbar fluid pressure even in case of a complete obstruction. Presumably, such a rise results from a rapid increase in the intra-abdominal and intrathoracic pressures, thus temporarily obstructing venous return from the spinal veins.

In acute lesions (fracture or dislocation of the vertebrae) the fluid below the point of obstruction may be normal in appearance. If the lesion producing the obstruction is of longer duration than 2 or 3 days, the lumbar fluid becomes xanthochromic and clots after withdrawal because of its high protein content (the Froin syndrome). Incomplete obstructions, even of slight degree, are characteristically associated with an increase of total protein—the amount depending upon the degree of compression.

The normal cerebrospinal fluid pressure in the horizontal position varies from 70 mm. to 200 mm. of fluid, the average normal pressure being about 130 mm. Pressures between 200 and 250 mm. are suspiciously high, and those above 250 mm. are definitely abnormal. Pathological states which are commonly associated with very high cerebrospinal fluid pressure are acute pyogenic meningitis, brain tumors, contusion and laceration of the brain from trauma, hemorrhage, both cerebral and meningeal, and brain abscess. Diseases frequently associated with a moderate increase of cerebrospinal fluid pressure are tuberculous and luetic meningitis, irritative meningitis, poliomyelitis, encephalitis, and uremia.

A lowered cerebrospinal fluid pressure is frequently observed in cases of head injuries, fainting or shock, and degenerative lesions of the nervous system where there is an actual diminution of neural substance. Certain cases of intractable headache are observed to have a very low fluid pressure, the cause of which has never been adequately explained.

LABORATORY TESTS.—Examination of the cerebrospinal fluid is necessary for the diagnosis of many diseases of the nervous system. The fluid has been subjected to almost every conceivable test in order to obtain information concerning the nature of the lesion in the nervous system. Many of these tests are of no practical concern, but the value of the information derived from others has greatly facilitated neurological diagnosis.

The all-too-common practice of "doing a spinal fluid Wassermann" without attempting to analyze the fluid further cannot be too strongly condemned. It simply means that the patient must be subjected again to the inconvenience of a lumbar puncture when he is seen by the neurological consultant, who will almost surely require the information derived from chemical and cytological tests.

Every specimen of fluid should be subjected to the following examinations routinely:

1. Color.
2. Cell count.

3. Globulin.
4. Total protein.
5. Colloidal gold curve.
6. Wassermann.

If there is an elevation in the number of cells, the following tests should be made in addition:

7. Staining of a centrifuged specimen for microörganisms.
8. Cultures—and, on certain occasions, animal inoculations.
9. Sugar.

1. There is no *color* to normal cerebrospinal fluid; it has the appearance of distilled water. In certain pathological conditions its appearance is changed. Purulent meningitis is almost always associated with a "milky," cloudy fluid, the degree of cloudiness depending upon the number of leucocytes present. In meningitis associated with poliomyelitis and encephalitis, however, the fluid may remain clear and colorless. A yellow tint to the fluid, xanthochromia, is produced by free hemoglobin in various stages of decomposition. Xanthochromic fluid is observed after old hemorrhage into the subarachnoid space from trauma, tumors, certain infections, and spontaneous rupture of blood vessels in or near the cerebrospinal fluid pathways. Fluids contaminated by fresh blood have a red and not a yellow tinge. In case of doubt as to the clear, colorless nature of the fluid, one should fill a test tube with tap water and compare it with the tube of fluid.

2. The *cell* count is perhaps the most important single examination of the cerebrospinal fluid. Furthermore, it is a test that requires care, experience, and a knowledge of the morphological characteristics of leucocytes. Perhaps the greatest confusion for the novice arises from his inability to differentiate between red blood cells and leucocytes, especially if there are only a few cells present. The author has found the following method of preparing the fluid for the counting chamber to be simple, useful and devoid of many sources of error:

Fill a white blood cell pipette with glacial acetic acid. Gently blow out the acid until no liquid is seen in the stem of the pipette. Draw the fluid into the pipette until the bulb is about one-fourth full. Allow to stand for 2 or 3 minutes. Then discard the first drop of fluid from the end of the pipette and apply the second and third drops to the counting chamber.

With this method, the fluid is counted undiluted, except for the volatile acetic acid left in the pipette. If the fluid contains a few red blood cells, they are either hemolyzed or badly crenated by the acid. Also, due to the action of the acid, the nuclear material of the leucocytes becomes very prominent, and a satisfactory differential count may be made from the counting chamber preparation.

An increase of cells signifies irritation or inflammation of the meninges. A predominance of lymphocytes usually indicates a non-pyogenic infection such as syphilis in one of its many forms, encephalitis, poliomyelitis, tuberculous meningitis, fungus infections, or lymphatic leukemia. A predominance of polymorphonuclear leucocytes indicates usually an infection with some pyogenic organism such as the meningococcus, Streptococcus, Staphylococcus, pneumococcus, or influenza bacillus. However, a predominance of polymorphonuclears may occur with pyogenic infections in the neighborhood of the meninges, as in mastoiditis or acute brain abscess, when no actual contamination of the meninges with an organism has occurred. Such conditions are usually spoken of as irritative meningitis. Also, certain chemical irritations of the meninges, such as the injection of air or lipiodol into the subarachnoid space, produce a high cell count with a predominance of polymorphonuclears.

3. The protein content of the cerebrospinal fluid consists of *globulin* and *albumin*. No simple test is available to determine the globulin content quantitatively. However, the qualitative methods give a reliable index to any significant increase in the globulin content. There is a marked increase in all acute infections of the meninges; in fact, any disorder which produces an elevation of the cell count also causes some increase in the amount of globulin. Globulin is increased in diseases of the nervous system other than those of inflammatory origin. In many degenerative lesions, such as multiple sclerosis, the

globulin is increased moderately. In certain tumors of the brain, particularly if they lie in close proximity to the cerebrospinal fluid pathways, the globulin is increased. Any neoplasm or other obstruction of the spinal canal produces in the spinal fluid below the obstruction marked increase of globulin. If an obstruction of this sort becomes complete or nearly so, the protein content of the fluid becomes excessively high, and when the fluid is exposed to air, spontaneous coagulation occurs. Such a fluid is xanthochromic and usually free of cells—the Froin syndrome.

4. Estimation of the *total protein* content of the cerebrospinal fluid is a quantitative test of great importance. In this test, the globulin and albumin fractions are estimated as one. In ordinary circumstances, there is a fairly constant 1:3 ratio between the globulin and total protein. Since the total protein is a quantitative one, more information may be obtained from it than from the qualitative globulin test, although an increase in either has the same significance. Not infrequently, the globulin test will be questionably positive, yet the total protein determination will show an unmistakable increase over normal. Furthermore, accurate determination of the protein content gives reliable information as to the progress of the inflammatory lesions, and it is especially helpful in determining the degree of spinal subarachnoid blockage. The significance of a rise in total protein is identical with that stated above for globulin.

5. The *colloidal gold curve* of Lange is useful in differentiating between certain organic diseases of the nervous system. Apparently, the changes in color of the gold solution observed in this test are due to union with certain protein radicals of the cerebrospinal fluid. As a matter of practical importance, the gold curve usually is normal unless there is an excess of protein present.

The characteristic types of curves are as follows:

(a) The normal curve   0000000000
(b) The luetic curve   1223100000

(c) The paretic curve   5555554310

(d) The curve often seen in brain tumor and tuberculous meningitis   0000123100

(e) The curve often seen in meningitis other than tuberculous   0000012334

Many variations from these characteristic types occur, and it is often impossible to classify an atypical curve. The test is most reliable in differentiating syphilitic infections of the nervous system, as they most frequently conform to their own type. However, a luetic or paretic type curve does not indicate syphilis unless the Wassermann reaction is also positive. A luetic curve is found frequently in fluid in which there is an excess of protein from any cause. A typical paretic curve with a negative Wassermann is frequently found in multiple sclerosis.

6. The *Wassermann reaction* should be done on all specimens of cerebrospinal fluid as a matter of routine. Not infrequently, the cerebrospinal fluid reaction is positive when the blood serum is repeatedly negative. The test is accurate in ninety to ninety-five per cent of all syphilitic infections of the nervous system. The presence of a positive spinal fluid Wassermann should not overshadow clinical evidence pointing to a different diagnosis, particularly brain tumor. Many patients with operable tumors have been robbed of every chance for recovery simply because they were so unfortunate as to have a positive spinal fluid or blood Wassermann.

7. When there is an elevation in the number of cells in the fluid, certain other studies should be made. A specimen of the fluid should be centrifuged and the sediment stained for microörganisms. In cases of purulent meningitis, this examination is of the utmost importance from the standpoint of treatment and prognosis. Pneumococci, streptococci, and staphylococci if present are usually in large numbers and are easily recognized. Meningococci, on the other hand, are often extremely difficult or impossible to find in the smear. In fact, so frequently is this the case, that a very satisfactory routine to follow, when

fulminating symptoms are present, is to start active treatment of the patient while the culture is incubating.

8. Needless to say, a culture should be made in every case of suspected meningitis. In certain instances, particularly when tuberculous meningitis is suspected, guinea-pig inoculation should be employed if the organisms cannot be identified unmistakably in the smear.

9. The *sugar* content of the cerebrospinal fluid is often helpful in differentiating between certain inflammatory lesions of the nervous system. In all pyogenic infections, the sugar content is markedly reduced. In certain cases of encephalitis, the sugar is increased in amount. In non-inflammatory conditions, the sugar content shows no significant change.

The reader is referred to Table II for an abbreviated summary of the cerebrospinal fluid changes found in the frequently encountered diseases of the nervous system.

TABLE II*

SUMMARY OF THE CEREBROSPINAL FLUID FINDINGS IN HEALTH AND DISEASE

Disease	Pressure: mm. of Spinal Fluid Horizontal Position	Rise on Jugular Compression	Appearance	Cells per cmm.	Protein mgm/100 cc.	Sugar mgm/100 cc.	Comment Heavy Type Indicates Findings Most Important in Differential Diagnosis
Normal: Lumbar	70–200	Prompt	Clear Colorless No Clot	0–5	15–45	50–75	Sugar values apply to fasting individuals with normal plasma values. Normal values for urea nitrogen: 5–20 mgs./100 cc. for non-protein nitrogen: 10–35 mgs./100 cc. Globulin usually parallels protein content. Gold sol reaction is so variable it has little diagnostic value except where indicated below.
Cisternal				0–5	10–25	50–75	
Ventricular				0–3	5–15	55–80	
"Bloody Tap" Normal Fluid	N	N	Bloody; Supernatant Clear	+	±	N	**Variation in amount of blood in different tubes. If** much blood present clot will form. **Supernatant fluid clear and colorless,** or pink if hemolysis has taken place; **never yellow.**
Subarachnoid or Ventricular Hemorrhage	+	N	Bloody; Supernatant Yellow	+	+	N	**All tubes equally bloody. Does not clot. Yellow tint to supernatant fluid within 4 hours after hemorrhage. This increases for 8–10 days until all red cells have disappeared.** White blood cells often increased in fluid; at first, polys; later, mononuclear cells. When blood disappears pressure becomes normal. If bleeding due to tumor, pressure remains high.
Acute Purulent Meningitis	+	N	Clear to Purulent Faint Yellow Clot +	+	+	Low	Sugar may be but slightly decreased at outset. Often falls rapidly to under 10 mgm. Meningococci and influenza bacilli found in smear and culture with difficulty; pneumococci, streptococci and staphylococci easily. Indol present in influenza meningitis.
Tuberculous Meningitis	+	N	Opalescent to Turbid Faint Yellow + **Delicate Fibrin Web**	+ Mononuclears	+	Decrease	**Progressive fall in sugar** (occasionally high at outset) Occasionally very early in disease and in infants polys predominate. Tubercle bacilli may be found in clot or sediment. Guinea pig inoculation positive.

* Most of the data in this table were copied from the charts of Fremont-Smith published in Arch. Neurol. & Psychiat., **27:** 691 (March) 1932.

TABLE II (*Continued*)

Acute Syphilitic Meningitis	+	N	Clear to Turbid Faint Yellow ± Fibrin Clot	+	+	N or Slightly Low	Wassermann reaction nearly always positive.
Acute Anterior Poliomyelitis	+	N	Slight Opalescence Rarely Turbid Faint Yellow ± Delicate Fibrin Web	+	Slight +	N or Slight Increase	In preparalytic stage polys may exceed 80%.—Rapid change to mononuclears. With gradual decrease in cells protein increases for two to three weeks.
Encephalitis Lethargica	N	N	N	N or Slight Increase No Polys	N or Slight Increase	N or Slight Increase	Sugar is normal unless blood sugar is elevated. Cell count rarely exceeds 60. Over 50% of cases have normal cell count. Protein increase when present is slight—rarely reaching 100 mgm/100 cc.
Acute Encephalitis (meningeal form)	+	N	N to Slightly Opalescent	+	Slight Increase	+	Cell count usually between 100 and 300 per cu. mm. Mononuclears 75 to 80% Polynuclears 20 to 25%.
Brain Tumor	+	N or delayed	N or Yellow	Rarely Increased	N or +	N or +	Pressure nearly always increased. Occasionally normal after catharsis or marked dehydration. See below.
Brain Abscess	+	See Brain Tumor	Clear and Colorless to Turbid Clot ±	+	Slight Increase	N or +	Pressure high. Polys nearly always present. Brain Abscess represents one form of "Aseptic Meningeal Reaction." Extradural abscess and lateral or cavernous sinus thrombosis give similar picture. The cell count may be only slightly increased or several thousand per c.mm. In the latter case distinguish from purulent (bacterial) meningitis by normal or only slightly lowered sugar value. In purulent meningitis the sugar is nearly always below 40 mgs per 100 cc. Subacute bacterial endocarditis with emboli to brain may cause increased pressure, cells (polys) and protein.
Subdural Hematoma	+	N	Yellow or N	N occasionally few red blood cells	N or Sl +	N	A yellow fluid under increased pressure with normal or only slightly increased protein rarely occurs in any other condition.
"Epilepsy"	N	N	N	N	N	N	Normal fluid. Protein occasionally slightly increased.

TABLE II (*Continued*)

Disease	Pressure: mm. of Spinal Fluid Horizontal Position	Rise on Jugular Compression	Appearance	Cells per cmm.	Protein mgm/100 cc.	Sugar mgm/100 cc.	Comment — Heavy Type Indicates Findings Most Important in Differential Diagnosis
Multiple Sclerosis	N	N	N	±	±	N	**A strong paretic or luetic gold sol reaction in presence of negative Wassermann reaction in patient not previously treated for syphilis is strong evidence of multiple sclerosis.**
Lead Encephalopathy	+	N	N or Slightly Yellow	+	N or +	N or +	Cells nearly always increased, occasionally up to several thousand—chiefly lymphocytes. Occasionally polys predominate especially in children. Pressure nearly always elevated. Lead is present in cerebrospinal fluid.
Uremia	+	N	N Occasionally Slightly Yellow	N or sl. +	N or +	+	**Urea and Non-protein nitrogen increased. Sugar high** because of hyperglycemia. Gold sol may show paretic curve. Occasionally cells or protein may be slightly increased and slight yellow color may be present.
Meningo-Vascular and Parenchymatous Syphilis	±	N Rarely delayed	N Rare Fibrin Clot	+	+	N	**Wassermann reaction nearly always positive in lumbar fluid, but may be negative in ventricular fluid. Gold sol reaction nearly always in paretic or luetic zone.**
Cerebral Arteriosclerosis and Arterial Hypertension	Usually Normal	N	N Occasionally Slightly Yellow	N or sl. +	N or +	N	**Pressure usually normal even with extreme arterial hypertension.** With cardiac decompensation and high venous pressure cerebrospinal fluid pressure will be high. Occasionally these cases have unexplained high intracranial pressure with choked disc and are extremely difficult to differentiate from brain tumor.
Cervical and Thoracic Herniations of the Nucleus Pulposus	N or Low	Delayed or Absent	N or Slightly Yellow	N	+++	N	Partial or complete block to the Queckenstedt test in about one-half of the cases.
Lumbar Herniations of the Nucleus Pulposus	N	N	N	N	++	N	No block demonstrated unless puncture performed below the level of the lesion. As 95% of these lesions occur at the level of the fourth and fifth lumbar interspaces puncture below the level of the lesion is usually not attempted.

TABLE II (*Continued*)

SPINAL SUBARACHNOID BLOCK (TUMOR, POTT'S DISEASE, MENINGITIS, ETC.)

Partial Block	Lumbar	N or Low	Delayed	N or Faint Yellow Clot Rare	±	+	N	Partial block is best demonstrated by combined cistern and lumbar puncture.
	Cisternal	N	Prompt	N	±	N	N	Pantopaque arrest, but some passes by the block.
Complete Block	Lumbar	Low or N	Absent	Colorless with slight clot, to deep yellow with massive coagulation	±	+++	N	Little fluid obtainable. Rapid drop in pressure to zero.
	Cisternal	N	Prompt	N Faint Yellow Color or Clot Rare	±	±	N	Cistern puncture not necessary to demonstrate block. Pantopaque completely arrested.
Tumor of Cauda Equina	Lumbar (below tumor)	Low	Absent or Delayed	Colorless with slight clot, to deep yellow with massive coagulation	N	+++	N	
	Lumbar (above tumor)	N	Prompt	Yellow or Colorless, Clot ±	N	++	N	
	Cisternal	N	Prompt	N Yellow Color or Clot Rare	N	±	N	
Original "Froin Syndrome"		Low or N	Absent	Deep Yellow Clear, Massive Coagulation	+	+++	N	See "Complete Spinal Subarachnoid Block"—above. Distinguish from late subarachnoid hemorrhage by high protein content.

PART III

ROENTGEN DIAGNOSIS

CHAPTER IX

ROENTGEN DIAGNOSIS*

Examination of the skull and spine by means of the x-ray is an important adjunct to neurological diagnosis. Moreover, through the medium of the x-ray, it is possible, after the injection of certain foreign substances into the confines of the skull and spinal canal, to localize accurately disorders of the nervous system which previous to the use of these methods would have remained obscure. Such diagnostic methods do not in any sense replace in importance a thorough neuroclinical study. They are laboratory procedures which have definite merit when thoughtfully applied.

Roentgen diagnosis will be considered under the headings of: (1) Plain films of the head and spine. (2) Air studies of the brain—ventriculography and encephalography. (3) Myelography.

(1-a) PLAIN FILMS OF THE SKULL

It must be remembered that shadows are cast upon the x-ray film only by substances which absorb the x-rays to a greater degree than the adjacent structures. The nervous tissue and coverings are of such uniform density that the shadows cast upon the film are completely wanting in detail. However, calcification, which normally occurs in the skull, pineal gland and occasionally in the falx cerebri, and which may abnormally occur in nervous tissue itself, casts shadows upon the film which are exact in detail and, consequently, important in diagnosis.

The technique involved in making x-ray films of the skull has been so refined by the use of fine focus tubes and the Bucky diaphragm, that it is now possible to produce negatives which show the minute structure of these calcified parts. Further-

* The author makes no attempt to deal fully with the principles of x-ray diagnosis as applied to neurology. Only a few elementary principles of the problem are indicated.

185

more, through the use of the stereoscopic apparatus, it is possible to produce films which, when studied, give a third dimension to the image. By means of a stereoscopic examination, it is
possible to examine the interior of the skull, both the inner
and the outer tables, the base, and such areas of calcification as
may occur normally or abnormally within the brain tissue
itself.

HEAD FILM TECHNIQUE.—The films are made on a flat
table with the patient in the horizontal position. A specially
devised fixation apparatus, developed by Dr. J. C. Bell, is

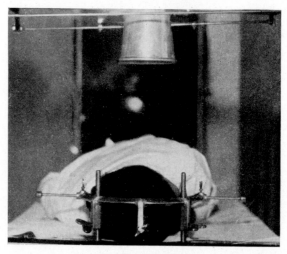

FIG. 60. Position of the patient, fixation apparatus, and x-ray
tube for making lateral stereoscopic films of the skull.

most useful for immobilization and accurate centering. Stereoscopic films are made in both lateral positions (Fig. 60), in
the anteroposterior and posteroanterior positions (Figs. 61, 62).
All exposures are made through the Bucky diaphragm.

Stereoscopic films in four positions are always desirable for
the part of the skull in closest contact to the film can then be
studied in minute detail. Furthermore, the position of any abnormal areas of calcification can thus be more accurately
localized.

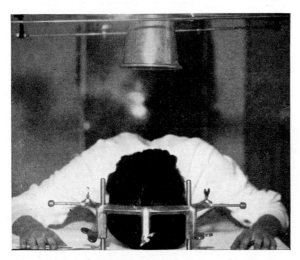

FIG. 61. Position of the patient, fixation apparatus, and x-ray tube for making posteroanterior stereoscopic films of the skull.

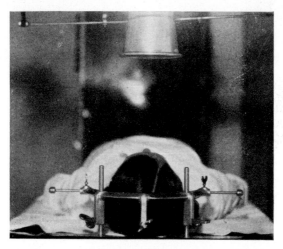

FIG. 62. Position of the patient, fixation apparatus, and x-ray tube for making anteroposterior stereoscopic films of the skull.

LANDMARKS AND MARKINGS.—It is desirable to establish a careful routine in examining a set of stereoscopic head films.

First. The cranial vault should be scrutinized closely for abnormal markings. On the inner table, the markings of the arterial channels are fairly constant in position and course. The grooves in the temporal bones in which the middle meningeal

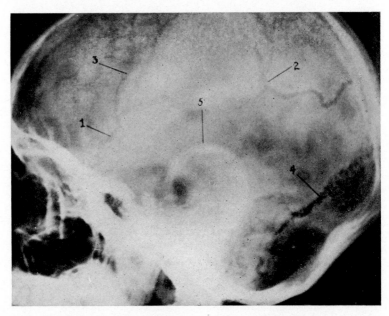

FIG. 63. Lateral view of a normal skull. 1. The channel of the middle meningeal artery. 2. Venous channels in the diploë of the skull. 3. The coronal suture. 4. The lambdoidal suture. 5. Shadow cast by the cartilage of the ear. Note the contrast between the channels of the meningeal artery and the diploic veins.

arteries lie are most important landmarks. The channels in the inner tables in which branches of these arteries lie can ordinarily be traced in the temporal, parietal and frontal bones (Fig. 63). Normally, the channels are the same size on each side. The vascular markings of the diploic vessels, i.e., those vessels that run between the outer and the inner tables of the skull, vary in prominence. The patterns of these diploic markings are quite dissimilar to those of the arterial channels in the inner table. They are venous channels, and their ramifications form an irregular pattern in contrast to the more or less regular course of the arterial channels. (Fig. 63).

In certain pathological conditions, particularly in slowly growing tumors arising from the meninges, the size of the

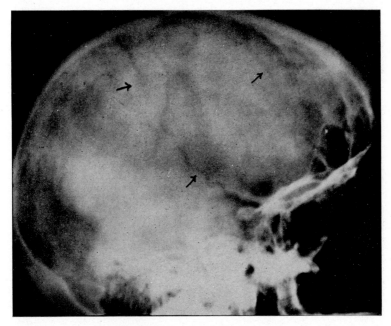

FIG. 64. Lateral views of the skull showing increased arterial markings in a case of parasagittal meningioma. Arrows indicate the channels of the anterior and middle meningeal arteries.

middle meningeal channel on the side of the tumor may be greatly increased. Furthermore, in neoplasms of this sort, abnormal arterial channels, which do not appear to be connected or continuous with the middle meningeal markings, frequently are seen in the inner table of the skull (Fig. 64).

Fractures of the skull are most commonly linear in form. They usually extend from the vault toward the base. Fracture lines are distinguished from arterial channels because they run a more regular course, are more sharply defined and frequently extend across vascular channels (Fig. 65). True linear fractures are never associated with depressed bone. Stellate frac-

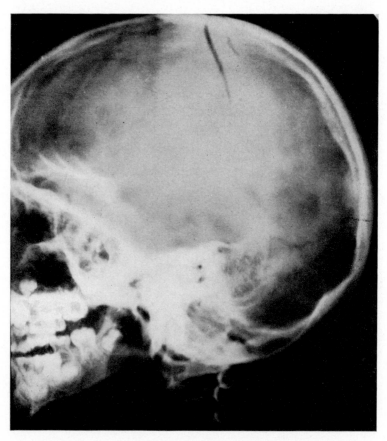

Fig. 65. Linear fracture of the skull. Note that the fracture line can be seen involving both tables.

tures, on the other hand, are frequently accompanied by displacement of bony fragments inward (Fig. 66).

Erosion of the overlying portion of the skull is seen frequently in tumors arising from the meninges. With small tumors, only the inner table may be eroded, but with large ones,

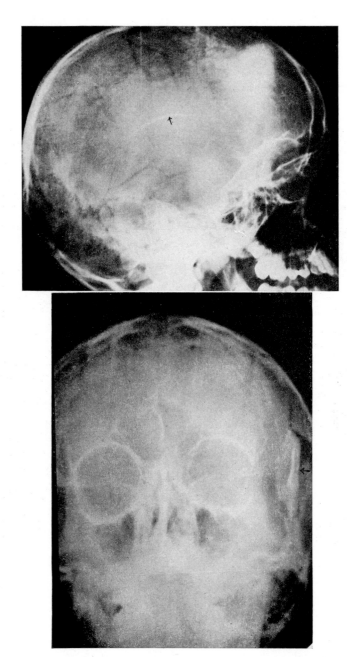

FIG. 66. Depressed fracture of the skull. In the lateral view, the arrows indicate a dense line which is produced by overlapping fragments of bone. Linear fractures without overlapping are seen below this area. A-P view shows inward displacement of the bony fragments.

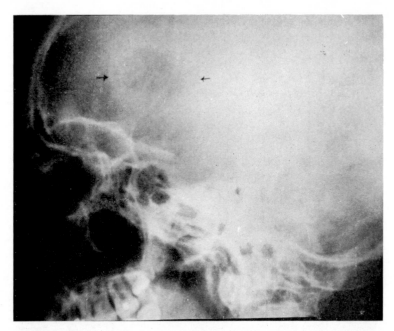

FIG. 67. Erosion of the skull from a meningioma arising from sphenoidal ridge. Note the faint markings on the inner table from the arteries supplying the tumor.

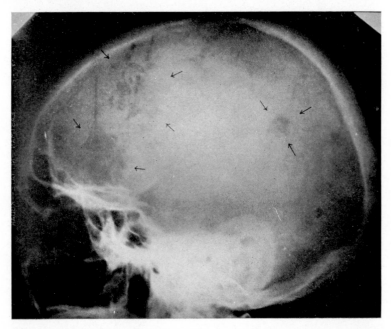

FIG. 68. Metastatic tumor of the skull from an adenocarcinoma of the prostate. Diploic venous channels are seen around the areas of destruction.

the erosion may involve both tables, and the tumor may form a bulging mass beneath the scalp (Fig. 67). Among the tumors which frequently metastasize to the skull and cause destruction are carcinomas of the breast, thyroid and prostate, hypernephromas and sarcomas (Fig. 68). The areas of destruction due to metastatic tumors are sharply outlined without evidence of abnormal vascular markings in the immediate vicinity

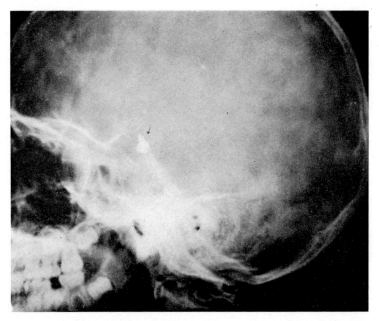

FIG. 69. Flaky calcification in the wall of a craniopharyngioma. Note marked destruction of the sella turcica and the pronounced digital markings.

of the erosion. With meningeal tumors, the erosion is usually accompanied by some increase in the arterial markings and often with bone production in the form of spicules.

Atrophy of the inner table, conforming to the convolutions of the brain, is seen frequently in cases of increased intracranial pressure. These *digital markings,* so-called, are seen normally in patients under the age of 10 years. After this age, an increase of these markings is at least suggestive of increased intracranial pressure. They are usually most prominent in the thin portions of the skull, particularly the squamous portion of the temporal bone. In cases of increased intracranial pressure of long standing, they may involve the entire inner table of the skull. (Fig. 69).

Absorption of bone adjacent to pacchionian granulations, which occurs most frequently at the vertex along the sagittal sinus—but may occur at any point in the inner table—is of no

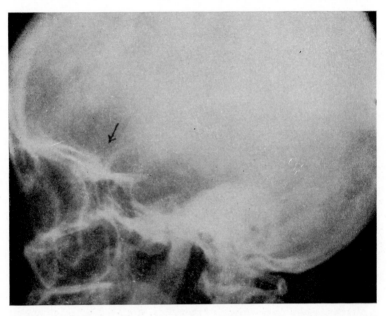

FIG. 70. Olfactory groove meningioma. Arrow indicates the "telltale" exostosis in the region of the cribriform plate. Note the calcification extending into the posterior ethmoidal cells.

clinical importance. The novice will, at first, find difficulty in distinguishing between the pacchionian impressions and pathological erosions of the skull. It is a safe rule to follow that any apparent erosion along the course of the sagittal sinus is almost surely due to a pacchionian body and, therefore, is without clinical importance.

An exostosis on either the inner or outer table of the skull may be of great clinical importance, because it frequently points to the site of an underlying meningioma. If exostoses of the inner table are associated with abnormal vascular markings, they almost surely indicate the presence of an underlying meningioma. Exostoses in the region of the cribriform plate are seen frequently in tumors arising from this area—the so-called olfactory groove meningiomas (Fig. 70).

A study of the posteroanterior films may give some idea of the condition of the accessory nasal sinuses but if a sinus in-

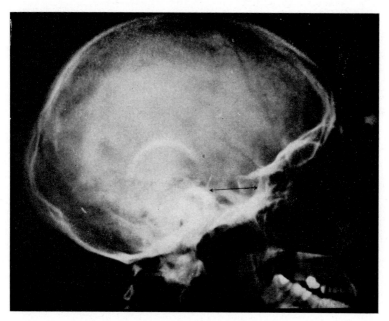

Fig. 71. Adenoma of the pituitary gland. Note tremendous expansion of the pituitary fossa, destruction of the base of the sella, and the thinning of the dorsum sellae.

fection is suspected, films should be made in the regular positions used in accessory nasal sinus examinations.

Second. The region of the sella turcica is especially important in neurological diagnosis, because of the frequency with which tumors occur in this region, and also because of the frequency with which this structure is destroyed or deformed due to tumors in other parts of the brain. Normally, the sella turcica is outlined by the *anterior clinoid processes* in front, the *dorsum sellae* behind, and the *thin floor* which projects into the sphenoid sinuses below. Tumors arising from the pituitary body destroy the contour of the sella in several ways. If the tumor arises within the sella turcica, there is gradual expansion of the entire fossa. The floor is depressed and the anterior and posterior confines are eroded or destroyed (Fig. 71). After pituitary

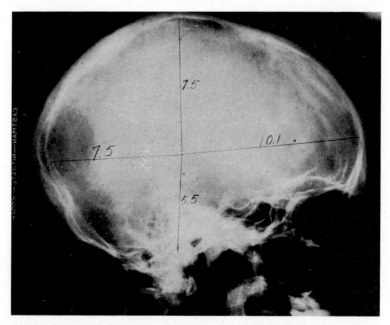

FIG. 72. Points on the skull from which measurements are taken to determine the location of the pineal gland.

tumors have attained considerable size, it is not infrequently found that all normal landmarks of the sella turcica are obliterated. In tumors arising above the sella turcica, the destruction may be confined to the clinoid processes and dorsum sellae. Tumors thus situated frequently contain flaky calcification, and their presence is shown by these deposits (Fig. 69).

Chronic increased intracranial pressure from any cause is frequently associated with distortions of normal landmarks of the sella turcica. This is usually manifest by erosion or destruc-

FIG. 73. Measurements of the distance from the pineal gland to the inner table of the frontal bone plotted against the sum of the distances from the pineal gland to the frontal bone and to the occiput. This sum is approximately equal to the greatest anteroposterior diameter of the skull. The pineal glands of normal skulls

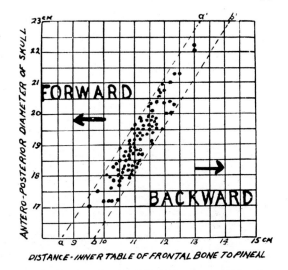

DISTANCE · INNER TABLE OF FRONTAL BONE TO PINEAL

were found to lie between the lines a–a' and b–b' which were considered to be the normal anteroposterior variation in position. (Vastine and Kinney)

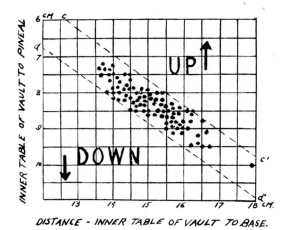

DISTANCE - INNER TABLE OF VAULT TO BASE.

FIG. 74. Measurements from the pineal gland to the inner table of the vault plotted against the sum of the distances from the pineal gland to the inner table of the vault and to the level of the base of the skull. This sum is approximately equal to the vertical diameter of the skull. The pineal glands of normal skulls were found to lie between the lines c–c' and d–d' which were considered to be the normal vertical variation in position. (Vastine and Kinney)

tion of the dorsum sellae, the clinoid processes, or displacement of these structures. Such deformities of the sella turcica are presumably due to distention of the third ventricle, thereby causing direct pressure upon these parts.

Third. Calcification of the pineal gland is

important as an aid in the localization of cerebral tumors. In the adult, it is calcified in at least 50 per cent of patients. Normally, the shadow cast by this structure lies exactly in the midline in the anteroposterior or posteroanterior films. A neoplasm, through pressure, may displace the shadow either lateralward,

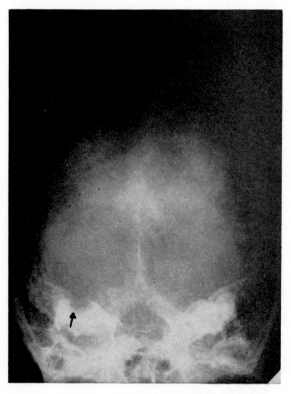

Fig. 75. Erosion of the petrous ridge from an acoustic neurinoma. Film taken in Towne's position.

upward, downward, forward, or backward, depending upon the position of the growth. In many instances, calcification of the pineal gland can be seen only in films made in the lateral positions. Vastine and Kinney have worked out an ingenious method for detecting pineal displacement from measurements on the

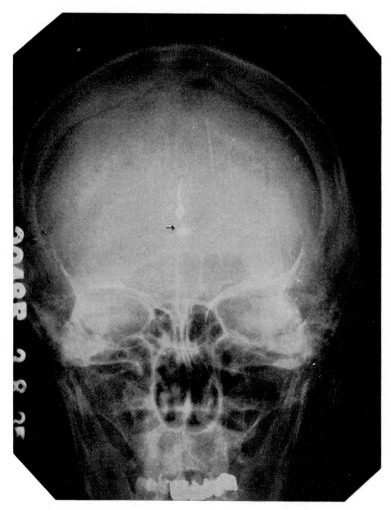

Fig. 76. Normal skull showing calcification in the falx. Arrow indicates the position of the calcified pineal gland.

lateral films. Their method is fully illustrated in Figs. 72, 73, and 74.

Fourth. Tumors arising around the petrous ridges of the temporal bone are frequently encountered. The most common ones are those neurinomas arising from the eighth cranial nerve—the so-called acoustic neurinomas. These neoplasms are of

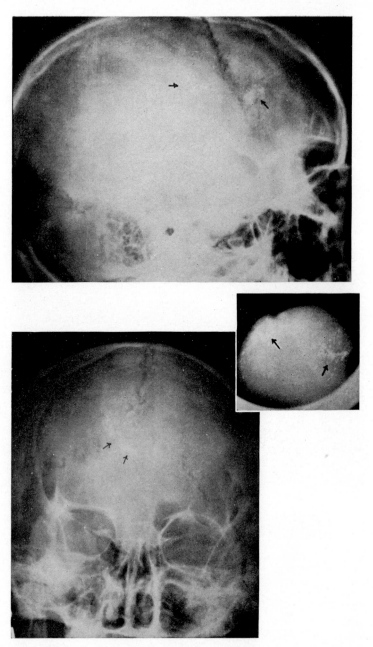

Fig. 77. Calcification in a right frontal meningioma. Lateral view shows multiple areas of calcification in the right frontal lobe. Posteroanterior view shows the relationship of the calcification to the midline of the skull. Insert shows an x-ray photograph of the tumor after surgical removal. Compare the size and position of the calcifications in the specimen with those shown on the lateral film.

slow growth; hence, as they gradually enlarge, destruction of the adjacent part of the petrous ridge takes place. Several positions for the study of the petrous ridges have been suggested. Perhaps the most satisfactory one is that of Towne's in which the outline of the ridges is brought into sharp relief (Fig. 75).

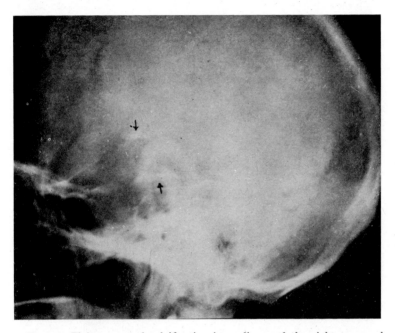

FIG. 78. Flaky areas of calcification in a glioma of the right temporal lobe. Note the characteristic shadow cast by the cartilage of the ear superimposed upon the denser calcification in the tumor.

Fifth. Abnormal areas of calcification in the brain substance are commonly seen in certain types of intracranial tumors; their presence and location may be determined with accuracy by careful study of the x-ray films. The only areas where deposits of calcium may occur without having clinical significance are the pineal gland, the falx cerebri and the choroid plexus (Fig. 76). Calcifications in these areas are recognized easily because of their characteristic locations.

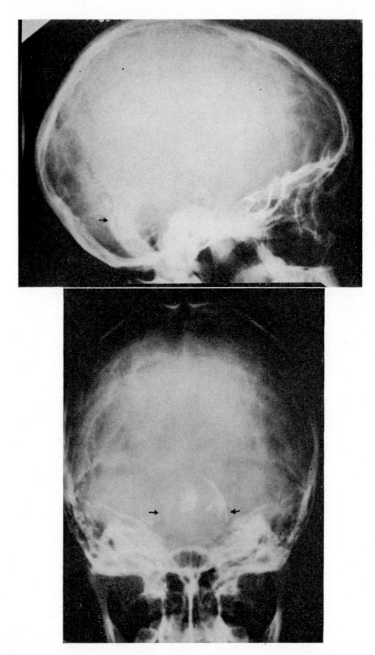

FIG. 79. Calcified glioma of the cerebellum. Lateral view shows the posterior wall of the tumor. P-A view shows the position of the tumor in relation to the midline of the skull.

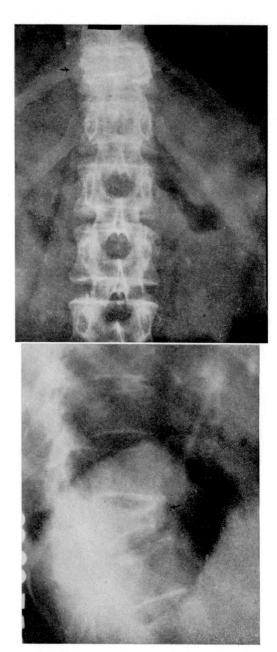

Fig. 80. Fracture of the 11th thoracic vertebra. A-P view shows some
narrowing of the 11th vertebra with decrease in the intervertebral space
between the 10th and 11th vertebrae. Lateral view shows marked crush-
ing of the body of the 11th thoracic vertebra with some kyphosis. This
case illustrates the value of studying spinal injuries in both anteroposterior
and lateral positions.

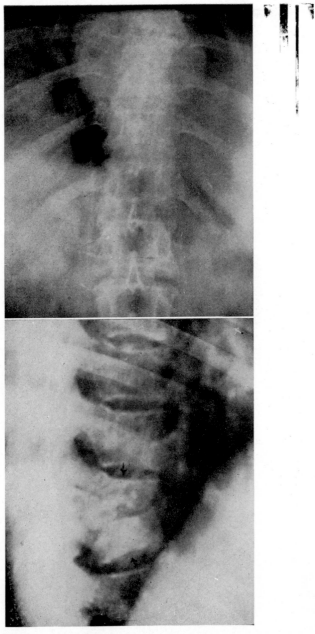

Fig. 81. Tuberculosis of the spine. Lateral view of lower thoracic spine, showing partial destruction of the bodies of the 9th and 10th vertebrae. The intervertebral space between the two vertebrae is entirely obliterated. A slight kyphosis has been produced. The A-P view shows the same destructive process involving the 9th and 10th vertebrae. In addition, the outline of a cold abscess can be seen.

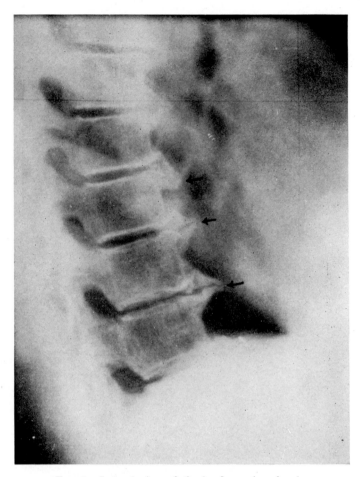

Fig. 82. Lateral view of the lumbar spine showing
advanced arthritic changes.

When a deposit of calcium is identified in other than these
locations, it points unmistakably to a pathological lesion, either
a neoplasm, an old hematoma, a vascular abnormality or a
tuberculoma (Figs. 77, 78, 79).

(1-b) Plain Films of the Spine

That part of the spine under suspicion because of the neurological findings should be subjected to a very careful x-ray ex-

amination. Stereoscopic films in the anteroposterior position
and a single film in the lateral position should be made. The
stereoscopic films permit a very careful examination of the

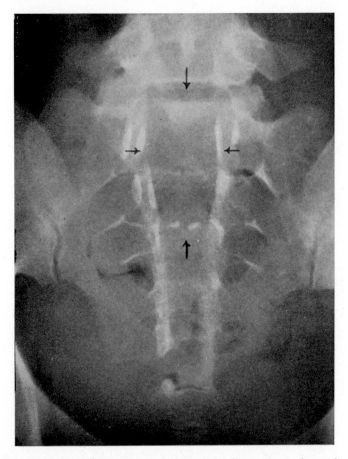

Fig. 83. Spina bifida occulta of the 5th lumbar and sacral vertebrae.
This patient suffered from motor and sensory paralysis of both feet due to
traction upon the sacral nerve roots.

laminae and processes of the vertebrae. The lateral film is
especially valuable in visualizing the vertebral bodies and intervertebral spaces. Fractures, dislocations, destructive lesions of
the bodies or intervertebral discs, and arthritic changes may be

shown more accurately on lateral films than on anteroposterior films (Figs. 80, 81, 82).

Incomplete fusion of the vertebral arches may or may not be of clinical importance. In the sacral vertebrae, defects in development of the arches frequently occur in adults. In the cervical spine, bifid spinous processes are normally found. In the fifth lumbar vertebra, the arch remains unclosed in perhaps 25 per cent of cases. In other regions of the spine, failure of the arches to fuse may be of considerable significance. If the arch is undeveloped and the neural canal is open posteriorly, the condition is called *spina bifida*. In many cases of spina bifida, there is an associated maldevelopment of the soft tissues over it. The meninges may extend into the soft tissues, forming a sac filled with cerebrospinal fluid—*meningocele*. Or the spinal cord elements may herniate into the sac forming a *meningomyelocele*. Frequently, however, no deformity of soft tissue can be demonstrated, yet the spina bifida may, because of cord involvement, be of great clinical importance—the so-called *spina bifida occulta* (Fig. 83).

Tumors arising within the neural canal may produce erosion of the pedicles or localized enlargement of one intervertebral foramen. Films taken in an oblique position are particularly valuable in showing such variances from the normal. Benign tumors arising within the canal may produce widening of the interpeduncular spaces.

Measurements of these spaces are made on the films taken in the anteroposterior position. Readings are made in millimeters and plotted on a chart as illustrated below:

Even though the interpeduncular measurements are increased in a localized area or over many vertebrae a diagnosis of intraspinal tumor should seldom be made unless there are definite destructive changes noted in the pedicles. The measurements may be increased in fractures of the vertebrae, spina bifida, or other developmental anomalies of the spine.

(2) AIR STUDIES OF THE BRAIN

Since Dandy's initial description (1918) of ventriculography

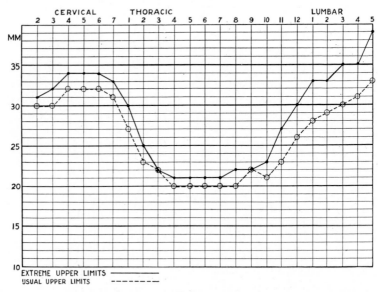

F<small>IG</small>. 84. The usual and the extreme size of the interpediculate space at each vertebral level in 100 x-rays of the normal spine. From Elsberg and Dyke, Bulletin of the Neurological Institute of New York, March, 1934.

and encephalography, air* studies of the brain have occupied a place of increasing importance in neurological diagnosis. Any lesion of the brain which encroaches upon or displaces the confines of the cerebrospinal fluid can be visualized directly or indirectly through the medium of x-ray films by replacement of all or part of the fluid with air. Like many other diagnostic procedures which, when viewed theoretically, should be 100 per cent efficient, air studies are subject to many pitfalls which make them, from a practical viewpoint, simply another adjunct to diagnosis—valuable when intelligently used, but pernicious when carelessly applied.

X-rays passing through the brain are absorbed equally by the

* Ordinary room air was the gas used originally by Dandy and in many clinics it is still preferred for both ventriculography and encephalography. Other gases have been used, notably oxygen, carbon dioxide and ethylene. In this clinic oxygen is used exclusively. However, the virtues of gases, other than air, are not easily demonstrated.

meninges, nervous tissue and the fluid which fills the ventricles; hence, no contrasting shadows are shown upon the photographic film. However, when the fluid spaces are filled with air, the rays are absorbed but slightly in their passage through the air, and a sharply defined contrasting shadow, conforming to the outlines of the fluid spaces, is shown upon the film. When the films are made stereoscopically, it is possible to view all of the cerebrospinal fluid system in which air replacement has occurred. If the total quantity of fluid has been replaced, the ventricular system, the subarachnoid spaces and the cisternae may be studied with remarkable accuracy.

The fluid within and around the brain may be replaced by air in two ways: First, by inserting a needle through an opening in the skull directly into the ventricle (ventriculography) and second, by withdrawal of fluid through a needle inserted into the spinal subarachnoid space (encephalography).

Ventriculography

Method.—By this procedure, an attempt is made to replace the fluid within the ventricular system with air. Needles are introduced into one or both lateral ventricles, the fluid withdrawn and replaced by air. The lateral ventricles may be tapped at a number of different points, but the one preferred is the posterior horn. A bilateral puncture is preferable; i.e., a ventricular canula is inserted into each lateral ventricle before the process of replacing the fluid with air is started. The procedure may be done by puncturing only one lateral ventricle, but less satisfactory filling of the ventricular system is likely to result.

Ten cubic centimeters of fluid are allowed to escape, and 9 c.c. of air injected. This process is repeated as long as fluid can be obtained. Care must be taken that the amount of air injected does not exceed the amount of fluid withdrawn, since air is expansible. The air should be filtered through sterile absorbent cotton.

When the air injection is completed, the patient is sent to

the x-ray room for stereoscopic films of the skull in the positions indicated.

Difficulties and Dangers of Ventriculography.—Interpretation of the ventriculograms is often the most difficult part of ventriculography. This is especially true if there has been incomplete filling of the ventricular system with air. In supratentorial tumors, when the intracranial tension is very high, it is often impossible to replace the fluid with air, because the ventricles collapse from tension after the fluid is withdrawn. In subtentorial tumors, it is often difficult to visualize the third ventricle. In such circumstances, the air studies may further complicate an already complicated diagnostic problem.

Ventriculography is a dangerous procedure, especially if performed by those unaccustomed to intracranial surgery. Unknown changes leading to cerebral edema may follow the sudden release of fluid from the ventricles, especially if the ventricular system is dilated. Air itself is an irritant, and produces an inflammatory reaction within the ventricles. The ventricular needle itself may pass through a soft tumor or injure the choroid plexus, thus causing a fatal hemorrhage.

Even in nonfatal cases, alarming reactions frequently occur. Headache and vomiting are of common occurrence. Drowsiness and even unconsciousness may supervene. These severe reactions may be avoided in many instances by the withdrawal of air from the ventricles after two or three hours. Fluid is reformed much more rapidly than the air is absorbed; hence, the greatest intracranial pressure is likely to occur in from 2 to 12 hours postoperatively. The intracranial pressure may also be reduced during this period by administration of hypertonic solutions intravenously or by mouth.

The best safeguard against fatal reactions is for the major operative procedure to follow immediately after completion of ventriculography. In this way, a large decompression is provided, and in many instances, the tumor which occasioned the air studies will have been removed. The air may be aspirated from time to time during the operation by tapping a lateral ventricle, or in case of a cerebellar tumor, by an indwelling

canula left in the ventricle during the entire operative procedure.

Many neurosurgeons have adopted the routine of resorting
to ventriculography only in the presence of a high degree of
choked discs, or when there is suggestive evidence of a posterior fossa lesion. In all other cases, when air studies are deemed

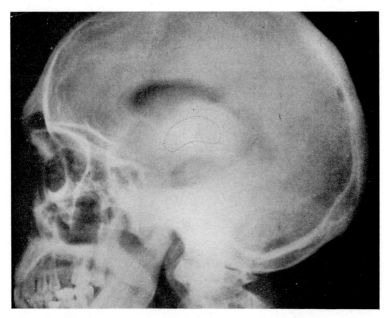

FIG. 85. Normal ventriculogram. Lateral view shows the outline of the
lateral ventricle with a very short posterior horn. The third ventricle is
incompletely filled with air and is outlined with dots to show its size and
position. The trephined opening in the skull is shown lateral to the midline
about 8 cm. above the external occipital protuberance. Note the normal
"clubbed" appearance of the anterior horns.

necessary, encephalography is employed. To this point of view
the author subscribes. In any circumstance, ventriculography
is never done unless, after careful neurological study, a localizing diagnosis cannot be made with certainty.

Interpretation of Ventriculograms.—One must be thoroughly familiar with the appearance of the normal ventricular

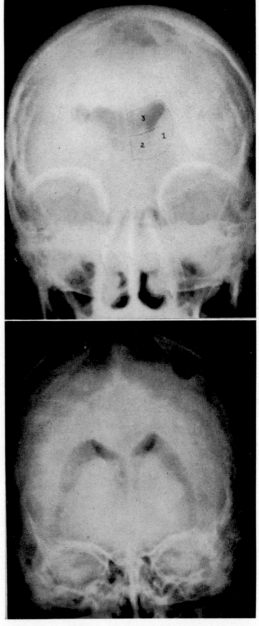

FIG. 86. Normal ventriculogram. A-P view shows the sagittal outline of the ventricles. On the left, the trephined opening overlaps the ventricular shadow. On the right, the ventricle is outlined by dots to illustrate the shadows cast by the different parts of the lateral ventricle when viewed anteriorly. 1. The shadow of the "clubbed" anterior horn. 2. The shadow of the ventricle in front of the thalamus. 3. This shadow is due to the total length of the upper portion of the body of the ventricle and, therefore, always appears darker than the rest of the shadows. P-A view shows the outline of the inferior horns in relation to the bodies of the lateral ventricles.

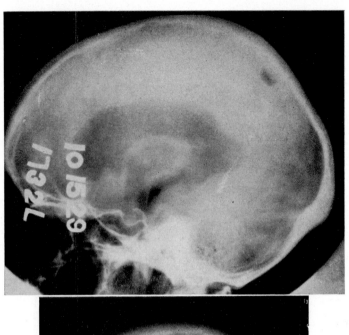

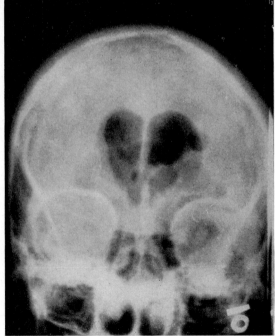

FIG. 87. Ventriculogram showing advanced internal hydrocephalus from a midline cerebellar tumor. Lateral view shows the dilated lateral and third ventricles. A-P view shows the symmetrical dilatation of the lateral ventricles and the large third ventricle.

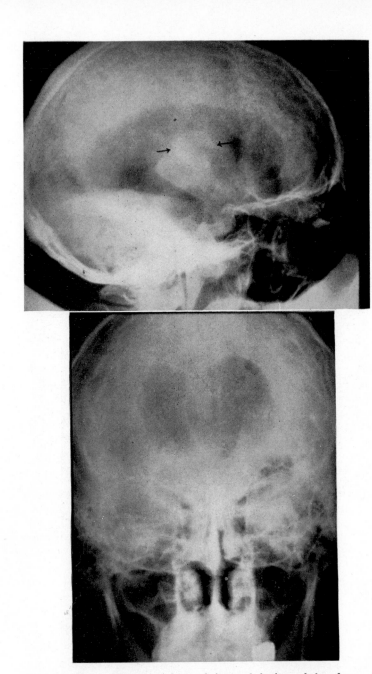

FIG. 88. Ventriculogram. Advanced internal hydrocephalus from obstruction of the 3rd ventricle by a tumor arising in the pineal gland. The lateral view shows the tremendous dilatation of the lateral ventricles. The arrows indicate the faint outline of the tumor projecting into the right lateral ventricle. No air in the third ventricle can be seen. The A-P view shows the symmetrical dilatation of the anterior horns with a complete absence of air in the 3rd ventricle.

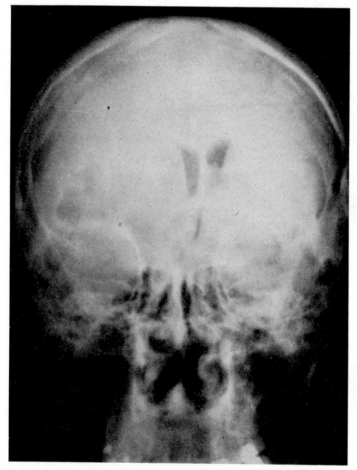

Fig. 89. Ventriculogram in a case of glioma of the left frontal lobe. Note the shifting of the ventricular system to the right, the slight deformity of the left lateral ventricle, and the displacement of the 3rd ventricle to the right.

system before attempting to interpret an abnormal one. The reader should study Figs. 85 and 86 in order to familiarize himself with the appearance of the normal ventricular system.

Expanding lesions of the brain cause two principal changes in the cerebral ventricles, symmetrical and asymmetrical alterations in their size, shape and position.

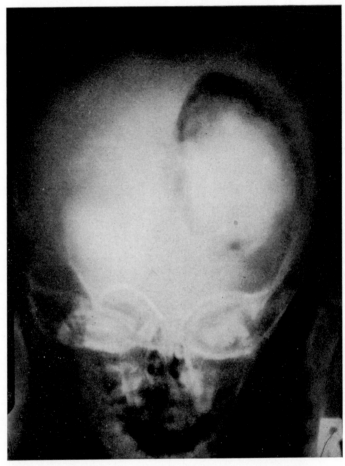

FIG. 90. Ventriculogram showing a large tumor (papilloma of the choroid plexus) in the right lateral ventricle. Note how the air completely encircles the tumor mass.

Symmetrical dilatation of the lateral ventricles may be produced by an obstruction to the exit of fluid at the third ventricle, the cerebral aqueduct or the fourth ventricle. The most common site of obstruction is at the fourth ventricle. When this occurs, in addition to the symmetrically dilated lateral ventricles, a dilated third ventricle may be seen (Fig. 87). The next most common site of obstruction is at the third ventricle.

If the obstruction is complete, no air can be made to enter it, and, therefore, it is not visualized in any position (Fig. 88). But if the obstruction is incomplete only the unobstructed portion can be visualized. Obstruction of the cerebral aqueduct occurs from inflammatory adhesions or from tumors of the pineal gland. The ventriculogram is of little use in differentiation between these obstructions and those of the fourth ventricle, unless the shadow of a pineal tumor can be seen protruding into one of the lateral or third ventricles.

Asymmetrical variations in the shape of the ventricles are usually due to lesions lying within the cerebral hemispheres lateral to the midline. The whole ventricular system may be shifted to the opposite side with a filling defect in the lateral ventricle on the side of the growth (Fig. 89), or the tumor outline may be clearly shown within the lateral ventricle (Fig. 90).

Encephalography

Replacement of the cerebrospinal fluid with air through a lumbar puncture needle is known as encephalography. After the air enters the spinal subarachnoid space, it floats upward into the cisterna magna. At this point, part of the air follows the cerebral subarachnoid space into the basal cisternae, and the remainder enters the fourth ventricle through the foramina of Luschka and Magendie, then by way of the aqueduct and the third ventricle it passes into the lateral ventricles. In this manner, all the fluid in the ventricular system and the cerebral subarachnoid space may be replaced with air. X-ray films made after such an injection show the outline of the entire cerebrospinal fluid system with remarkable clearness.

Method.—The patient should have the usual preoperative preparation. Some form of basal anesthesia may be used as the procedure is attended with considerable discomfort.

The patient is placed in a sitting position preferably in a specially designed chair that facilitates not only the spinal puncture but taking of x-ray films in the upright position. A simple inexpensive chair, used in this clinic for many years, is illustrated in Fig. 91.

Lumbar puncture is performed in the usual manner. After 10 c.c. of fluid have been collected, a similar amount of air is injected. It is desirable to filter the air (or other gas) through

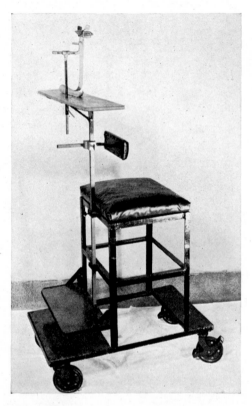

FIG. 91. Encephalogram chair. (J. C. Bell, *American Journal of Roentgenology and Radium Therapy*, Vol. XLII, No. 2, August, 1939.)

dry sterile cotton to reduce the danger of contamination from air borne microörganisms. After the replacement has reached 40 c.c. a preliminary lateral film of the skull is made without changing the position of the patient. Examination of the film reveals whether or not air has entered the ventricular system. If gas is found in the ventricles and the basal cisternae, 30 to 40 additional cubic centimeters of fluid are replaced with air.

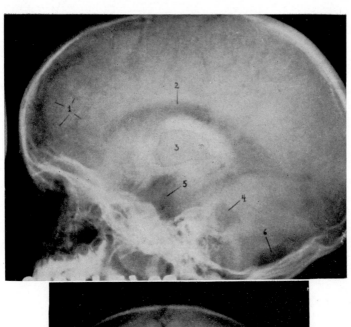

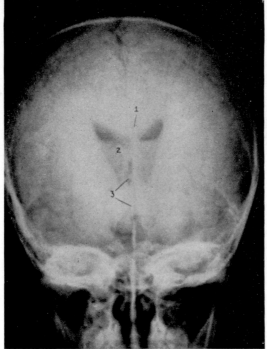

FIG. 92. A normal encephalogram. Lateral view shows: 1. Air in the cortical convolutions (cortical markings). 2. Lateral ventricle filled with air. 3. Third ventricle partially filled with air. 4. Fourth ventricle filled with air. 5. Chiasmatic cistern distended with air. 6. Cisterna magna partially filled with air. A-P view shows: 1. Air above the corpus callosum. 2. Lateral ventricles filled with air. 3. Third ventricle.

If no air has entered the ventricles the replacement should continue until all of the fluid has been exhausted. In about 5 per cent of patients filling of the ventricles will not occur. If a tumor is suspected the ventricles should be visualized at a later date by ventriculography.

Since in most instances there will have been incomplete replacement of fluid with air it is desirable to produce x-ray films in a variety of positions. Air, being lighter than fluid, will float on the surface of the fluid levels in the ventricles. Therefore, in studying the anterior part of the ventricular system a lateral film is made with the forehead up. To study the posterior system a lateral film is made with the forehead down. To study the superior portions of the ventricles a lateral film is made in the upright position. To study the ventricular system in the sagittal planes films are taken in the anteroposterior and posteroanterior positions. The positions desirable, therefore, for a complete encephalographic study are as follows:

(1) Stereoscopic films with the patient horizontal in the anteroposterior position, care being taken that the head is kept straight. (2) Lateral stereoscopic films in the upright position. (3) A single lateral film in the horizontal position with the forehead up. (4) A single lateral film in the horizontal position with the forehead down.

Films made in this manner show all parts of the ventricular system well distended with air—the subarachnoid space and the basal cisternae.

Reactions.—Headache is severe for the first 12 hours and ordinarily persists with gradual abatement for 2 or 3 days. Nausea, vomiting, and profuse sweating during the injection and for a few hours thereafter are of almost constant occurrence. Bradycardia of moderate degree is frequently observed. Reactions more severe than these are experiencd occasionally. If the contraindications are observed, encephalography is a much less dangerous procedure than ventriculography.

Contraindications.—The chief contraindications to encephalography are:

1. High degree of choked discs.

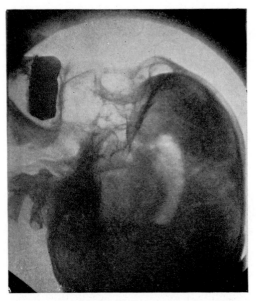

FIG. 93. A normal encephalogram. Lateral view with the forehead up. Note well distended portion of the lateral ventricles.

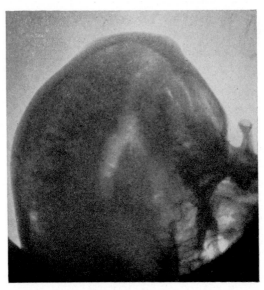

FIG. 94. A normal encephalogram. Lateral view with the forehead down. Note well distended posterior portion of the lateral ventricles.

2. Evidence of a lesion in the posterior fossa of the skull.

3. Evidence of an active inflammatory lesion of the meninges.

The same explanation prevails for the first two contraindications as have been previously recorded as contraindications to lumbar puncture (page 162). The third contraindication makes it desirable to perform lumbar puncture studies with analysis of the fluid before resorting to encephalography.

Indications.—Obscure neurological disorders in which an expanding lesion of the brain is a part of the differential diagnosis can usually be clarified by encephalographic studies.

All epileptics, whether they show localizing neurological signs or not, should be subjected to encephalography. If this procedure is made a routine in the investigation of the epileptic patient, many surgical lesions will be demonstrated and many otherwise hopeless cases will be benefited. Furthermore, the introduction of air into the cerebrospinal fluid spaces has some unexplained beneficial effect upon the number and severity of the seizures in some epileptic patients.

In cases with persistent headache from cerebral trauma, introduction of air into the subarachnoid space often has a beneficial therapeutic effect. In certain selected patients whose headaches are intractable to conservative measures an encephalogram is indicated not only for more accurate diagnosis but for the probable therapeutic effect.

Interpretation of Encephalograms.—The chief value of encephalography over ventriculography lies in the fact that it renders visible the cerebral subarachnoid spaces and the basal cisternae. If proper filling has occurred, the important sulci of the brain, the outlines of the corpus callosum and of the tentorium cerebelli can be visualized (Fig. 92).

The interpretation of ventricular deformities is the same as described in the section on ventriculography (page 209).

(3) MYELOGRAPHY

Visualization of the spinal subarachnoid space has been

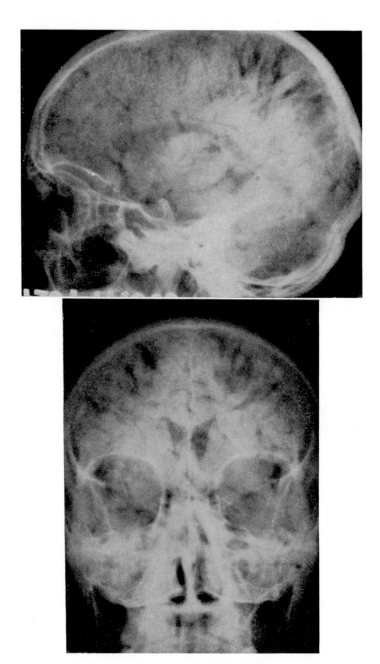

Fig. 95. Encephalogram in a case of advanced idiopathic epilepsy. Note the tremendous increase in the amount of cortical air with relatively little dilatation of the ventricular system.

accomplished generally by the use of three contrast media: (1) Lipiodol. (2) Thorotrast. (3) Air.

Lipiodol is in many respects a satisfactory myelographic medium. However, if the material is not removed, its tell-tale shadow persists more or less indefinitely. It can be removed, but the removal is attended with difficulties and at best is often incomplete.

Thorotrast gives excellent radiographic detail, and interpretations can be made with great accuracy. Thorotrast can be removed completely by continuous spinal drainage. However, there are many objections to its use, not the least of which is the time consuming procedure of continuous spinal drainage.

Air myelography is used more universally than any of the three, because air is absorbed and leaves no demonstrable x-ray evidence of its use. The headache caused by the attending meningeal irritation is often severe and incapacitating. The gas shadows, with highly refined radiographic technique, are subject to fairly accurate interpretations. However, in many instances, the radiographic diagnosis is presumptive and often equivocal.

A new myelographic medium is now available which combines the desirable qualities of lipiodol and thorotrast and is more easily removed by aspiration. If a few drops are left, they are absorbed within a few weeks. The material is *Pantopaque* and is the contribution of Dr. Stafford L. Warren, Professor of Roentgenology, University of Rochester (N.Y.) School of Medicine, and Dr. William Strain of the Eastman Kodak Company.

Indication for Myelography.—Pantopaque (ethyl iodophenylundecylate) injected into the spinal subarachnoid space is a valuable aid in demonstrating the exact level of an intraspinal lesion. The probable presence of such a lesion should have been determined by the clinical study, and only in those cases where neurological signs are not sufficiently clear-cut for accurate anatomical localization is the use of Pantopaque indicated.

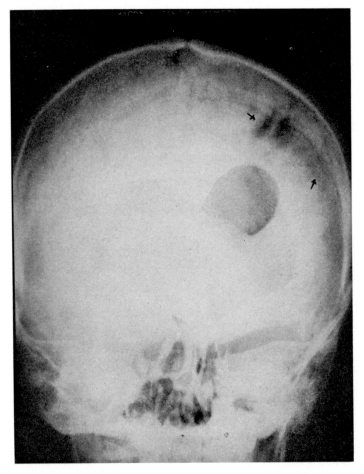

Fig. 96. Encephalogram in a case of jacksonian epilepsy. Arrows indicate the localized area of cortical atrophy. Note the unilateral dilatation of the contiguous ventricle with pulling of the ventricular system toward the diseased area.

Methods of Injection.—Pantopaque may be injected into the subarachnoid space either in the lumbar region or at the cisterna magna. The former injection site is preferable because of the simplicity and safety of lumbar puncture as compared with cisternal puncture. Only in exceptional instances is more information obtained from the roentgenological study when the oil is injected into the cisterna magna.

Surgical lesions involving the neural canal from the level

of the first cervical vertebra to the second lumbar vertebra inclusive (the space occupied by the spinal cord) usually encroach sufficiently upon the subarachnoid space to produce some degree of subarachnoid block. The *presence* of such a block can usually be demonstrated by the Queckenstedt test. However, the *location* of the block, whether partial or complete, may be difficult to determine from the clinical data. In these circumstances Pantopaque studies will demonstrate accurately the site of the lesion.

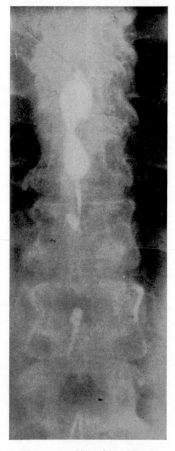

FIG. 97. Lumbar Pantopaque injection showing the indentation of the Pantopaque column due to a meningioma at the level of the 11th thoracic vertebra. There was an incomplete subarachnoid block as shown by the Queckenstedt test.

The patient is placed prone on the tilting fluoroscopic table with a small pillow beneath the abdomen. Lumbar puncture is done in this position, the needle being inserted distal to the 4th or the 5th lumbar spinous process. The puncture may be done below the 3rd spinous process, but at this level subsequent removal of the Pantopaque is more difficult. Spinal puncture in the face down position is as simple when one is accustomed to it as in the conventional position. One must be careful to keep in the midline and to insert the needle millimeter by millimeter after the ligamentum flavum is encountered. As soon as spinal fluid is obtained, the needle is inserted further about two millimeters and three cubic centimeters of Pantopaque injected. A stylet is then placed in the needle and the whole field covered with a sterile towel. The patient is now ready for fluoroscopy.

Pantopaque, being of low viscosity, is easily balanced at the desired level in the spinal canal by tilting the fluoroscopic table. Pantopaque, being heavier than spinal fluid, always seeks a dependent position in the subarachnoid space. As the column passes upward or downward to the desired level, spot films are made. When suspicious defects are encountered, oblique or lateral films (made with a portable unit) may be

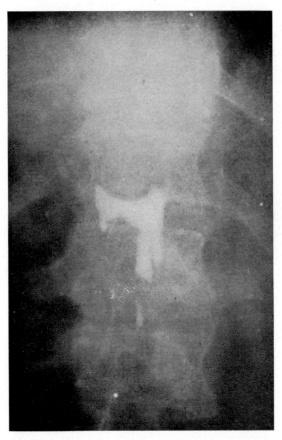

Fig. 98. Lumbar Pantopaque injection, showing complete arrest with "cap" formation at the 12th thoracic vertebra. The tumor was a neuro-fibroma.

made. Once the lesion is demonstrated and spot films of all suspected areas recorded, the column of Pantopaque is balanced at the point of the needle by tilting the table to the desired position. The needle is introduced about two millimeters further in order that aspiration may be accomplished as close to the anterior wall of the spinal canal as possible. A syringe is then attached and *gentle* aspiration begun. If the column has been carefully placed at the point of the needle, pure Pantopaque will be obtained and almost the entire amount may be recovered before fluid begins to bubble through the oily mixture. When spinal fluid appears, the syringe should be detached, the stylet reinserted and again the patient fluoroscoped to collect what remains of the Pantopaque around the point of the needle.

The whole examination, when one is experienced, requires but fifteen to twenty minutes including the injection and removal of the drug.

Spot films made with a grid show remarkably accurate detail. The dural sleeves and the axillary pouches are accurately outlined in most instances, and not infrequently the whole course of the nerve root may be shown at each level.

Myelography with Pantopaque, like myelography with other media, should not be attempted soon after a diagnostic lumbar puncture, certainly not until at least a week or ten days have elapsed. The continuous fluid drainage through the needle hole in the arachnoid often produces sufficient subdural fluid to make another subarachnoid puncture difficult or impossible. This is the most frequent cause of subdural and extra-arachnoid injections and, of course, when it occurs the myelograms are useless for interpretation. No untoward reactions are to be expected if the drug is removed immediately following the examination. Should, for any reason, removal not be complete, no greater reaction occurs than if lipiodol were used.

X-ray Interpretations: (a) **No obstruction.**—In this circumstance the Pantopaque column flows freely with any change of position of the patient. If the head is lowered quickly the column traverses the subarachnoid space into the cervical region with slow steady progress. When the position is reversed the opaque column progresses downward into the sacral sac.

(b) **Partial Block.**—When partial blocking of the spinal subarachnoid space occurs, the Pantopaque will be seen to approach this area and be temporarily arrested; a small stream will then pass around the obstruction, and gradually the entire mass will proceed in its ascent or descent in the canal (Fig. 97). Partial blocks may occur in: (1) Intramedullary tumors; (2) extramedullary tumors; (3) chronic inflammatory lesions of the meninges and spinal cord; (4) extradural abscesses; (5) primary or secondary disease of the vertebral bodies or arches with encroachment upon the neural canal; (6) lesions of the intervertebral discs.

In chronic inflammatory lesions of the spinal meninges, a characteristic myelogram is frequently seen. The column is broken up into many small masses, some of which gradually

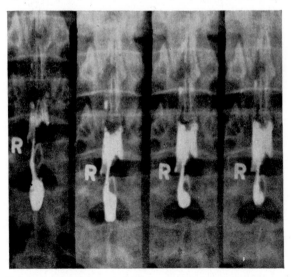

FIG. 99. Lumbar Pantopaque injection. Serial films showing gross filling defect due to a large herniated nucleus at the fourth lumbar interspace.

coalesce and continue the ascent or descent, while others are permanently arrested in the areas where there are adhesions.

(c) **Complete block.**—When the opaque column encounters a complete obstruction in the spinal subarachnoid space, it forms a distinct "cap" about the adjacent margin of the obstructing lesion. Complete obstructions are characteristically

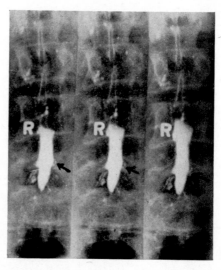

Fig. 100. Lumbar Pantopaque injection. Serial films showing obliteration of the left axillary pouch at the fifth lumbar interspace by a lateral herniation of the nucleus pulposus.

seen in patients with intradural tumors, particularly meningiomas and neurofibromas (Fig. 98).

(d) **Myelographic Defects in Lesions of the Cauda Equina.**—The most common and important lesion in this region is rupture of the intervertebral disc with herniation of the nucleus pulposus. Ninety-five per cent of these lesions occur at the fourth and fifth lumbar interspaces. The characteristic deformity at either interspace is: (1) A gross defect in the column as it passes over the ruptured disc (Fig. 99). (2) Obliteration, elevation or depression of the axillary pouch of the spinal nerve root due to a lateral herniation of the nucleus pulposus (Fig. 100).

INDEX

INDEX

Abdominal reflexes, 137
Abducens nerve, 32
Acoustic nerve, 47
Acuity of vision, 19
Adiadokokinesis, 96
Afferent neurons, 101, 102, 131
Air studies of the brain, 207
Ankle-clonus, 145
Ankle-jerk (Achilles'), 144
Anosmia, 15
Aphasia, 70
    motor, 70, 75
    sensory, 81
Aqueduct of Sylvius, 154
Arachnoid, 156
Arachnoidal villi, 158
Astereognosis, 77, 78
Asthenia, 91
Asynergy, 94
Ataxia, 92, 94
Atrophy of muscles, 121
Aura, 77, 78
Auscultation of head, 13

Babinski sign, 69, 138
Bárány test, 52
Betz cells, 65
Biceps reflex, 141
Bladder (urinary) disturbance, 125
Blind spot, 18
Broca's area, 70
Brown-Séquard syndrome, 117

Calcarine fissure, 78
Caloric test (Bárány), 52
Cauda equina, 99
Cerebellum, 89
    anatomy of, 89
    physiology of, 90
Cerebral aqueduct, 154
Cerebral hemispheres, 59
    corpus striatum, 82
    frontal lobe, 61
    motor speech area, 69

occipital lobe, 78
parietal lobe, 76
prefrontal area, 62
premotor area, 68
temporal lobe, 79
true motor area, 63
Cerebrospinal fluid, 153
    absorption of, 158
    cells, 174
    circulation of, 159
    color, 174
    composition of, 161
    formation of, 157
    functions of, 159
    protein, 176
Cerebrospinal fluid dynamics, 169
Cerebrospinal fluid in health and disease, 179
Cerebrospinal fluid pressure, 168, 169
Cerebrospinal fluid spaces, 153
Chaddock, 139
Choked discs (papilloedema), 28, 98
Choroid plexus, 155
Cisternae, subarachnoid, 156
Cochlear nerve, 47
Colloidal gold curve of Lange, 176
Conjugate deviation, 36
Contraindications to lumbar puncture, 162
Convulsions, 9
    grand mal, 9
    jacksonian, 10, 73
    psychomotor, 10
    sensory, 10
Coördination, 92
Corpus callosum, 60
Corpus striatum, 60, 82
Corticospinal tract, 65
    lateral, 65, 105
    ventral, 65
Cracked-pot resonance (Macewen's sign), 12
Cremasteric reflex, 137

233

This Book

PRACTICAL
NEUROLOGICAL
DIAGNOSIS

THIRD EDITION, SECOND PRINTING

was set, printed and bound by The Collegiate Press of Menasha, Wisconsin. The cover design is by the Fox Studio of Springfield, Illinois. The type face is 11 on 13 Linotype Old Style No. 7. The type page is 24 x 42 picas. The text paper is 60 pound White Wisconsin Enamel. The jacket is Linweave Text, Antique Finish. The binding is Interlaken-Vellum De Luxe T58.

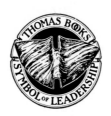

With THOMAS BOOKS careful attention is given to all details of manufacturing and design. It is the Publisher's desire to present books that are satisfactory as to their physical qualities and artistic possibilities and appropriate for their particular use. THOMAS BOOKS will be true to those laws of quality that assure a good name and good will.